Treatment-Resistant Bipolar Disorder

Stavroula Rakitzi • Polyxeni Georgila

Treatment-Resistant Bipolar Disorder

Evidence-based Pharmacotherapy, Cognitive Behavioral Psychotherapy and Rehabilitation

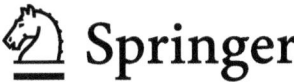 Springer

Stavroula Rakitzi (iD)
Clinical psychology and cognitive
behavioral psychotherapy
Private practice
ILISION 34 15771, Athens, Greece

Polyxeni Georgila (iD)
Psychiatry and cognitive behavioral
psychotherapy
Private practice
ILISION 34 15771, Athens, Greece

ISBN 978-3-031-59000-9   ISBN 978-3-031-59001-6   (eBook)
https://doi.org/10.1007/978-3-031-59001-6

This Springer imprint is published by the registered company Springer Nature Switzerland AG
The registered company address is: Gewerbestrasse 11, 6330 Cham, Switzerland

If disposing of this product, please recycle the paper.

This book is devoted to all the people with bipolar disorder and treatment-resistant bipolar disorder; to my patients with treatment-resistant bipolar disorder; to my parents and my family; to my colleague Polyxeni Georgila; and to Prof. Dr. Annette Schröder, my supervisor in my Ph.D. studies at the University of Koblenz-Landau, Germany.

Stavroula Rakitzi

This book is devoted to all the people with bipolar disorder and treatment-resistant- bipolar disorder; to my patients with treatment-resistant bipolar disorder; to my three daughters and to my sisters; to my parents; to my mentor Prof. E. Garelis; and to my colleague Stavroula Rakitzi.

Polyxeni Georgila

Preface

This book is about the modern and evidence-based interventions in treatment-resistant bipolar disorder that are being executed these days.

Furthermore, this book presents a modern point of view from us with respect to the therapy of treatment-resistant bipolar disorder—a new long-term recovery-oriented treatment as a combination of pharmacotherapy and cognitive behavioral therapy and rehabilitation.

This manual presents our clinical experience with treatment-resistant bipolar disorder. This subcategory of individuals with bipolar disorder faced numerous issues. So, it is exceptionally critical to have a conversation about a new point of view regarding the therapy of this subgroup. Our new recovery-oriented model guarantees a new beginning regarding therapy for people with treatment-resistant bipolar disorder and their families.

The mental health experts can, moreover, be propelled by our model in their own clinical practice.

The clinical psychiatrists, clinical psychologists, cognitive behavioral psychotherapists, students of psychology and medicine, and researchers can benefit as readership from this manual.

Athens, Greece   Stavroula Rakitzi
Athens, Greece   Polyxeni Georgila

Introduction

Treatment-Resistant Bipolar Disorder: Evidence-Based Pharmacotherapy, Cognitive Behavioral Psychotherapy and Rehabilitation presents an inclusive book about one of the most troublesome chronic mental health disorders, treatment-resistant bipolar disorder. Evidence-based treatments for treatment-resistant bipolar disorder, such as pharmacotherapy, cognitive behavioral psychotherapy, and rehabilitation, will be analyzed. A new recovery-oriented model for treatment-resistant bipolar disorder will be proposed. This book may be a valuable manual for experts, such as clinical psychiatrists, clinical psychologists, cognitive behavioral psychotherapists, and researchers, as well as students of psychology and medicine.

Acknowledgments

We are thankful to all of our patients with bipolar disorder and treatment-resistant bipolar disorder, who have participated in our treatments. We are also thankful to Dr. Sylvana Freyberg from Springer Nature and of course to Springer Nature.

Ethics Approval We adhere to the ethical standards of the 1964 Declaration of Helsinki and its subsequent alterations. We have included a statement that consent for publication was obtained from the participating individuals.

Competing Interests We declare that we have no competing financial or nonfinancial interests in connection with the content of this book.

About this Book

Treatment-resistant bipolar disorder presents one of the most difficult mental health disorders, which is associated with a high possibility of relapse, repetitive hospitalizations, suicidal behavior, and interpersonal problems.

This book focuses on treatment-resistant bipolar disorder, its clinical characteristics, and evidence-based treatments—pharmacotherapy, cognitive behavioral psychotherapy, and rehabilitation.

A new long-term recovery-oriented therapy for treatment-resistant bipolar disorder will be displayed.

Each chapter starts with an abstract, followed by learning objectives, an introduction, the main text, discussion, conclusions, revision questions, and a bibliography. The learning objectives and revision questions stimulate the learning of the readership. It can also contribute to the enhancement of the educational process in workshops and courses.

Dr. Stavroula Rakitzi
Dr. Polyxeni Georgila
Athens, Greece
January 2024

Contents

About the Authors

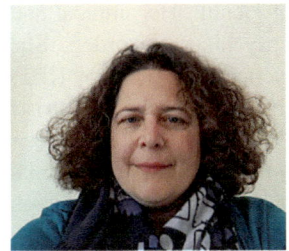

Stavroula Rakitzi completed her studies in psychology at the Georg-August University of Göttingen in Germany. She has the European Diploma in Psychology. She has completed her training in cognitive-behavioral psychotherapy in Athens according to EABCT criteria. Furthermore, she completed her Ph.D. in clinical psychology and adult psychotherapy at the University of Koblenz-Landau in Germany. Since 2001, she has worked as a Diplompsychologist and qualified cognitive-behavioral psychotherapist in private practice. She has been promoting Integrated Psychological Therapy (IPT) for individuals with schizophrenia since 2006 in Greece. She is a lecturer in cognitive behavioral therapy and in IPT at her private practice in Athens, Greece. Furthermore, she developed the IPT postgraduate program for psychologists and psychiatrists in Greece, trained in CBT. Likewise, she participated in many national and international conferences as a speaker and authored articles in Greek and international journals and books.

Furthermore, she is the author of the Springer Nature book *Clinical Psychology and Cognitive-Behavioral Psychotherapy. Recovery in Mental Health*. She is the editor of the Greek book *Intervention in Schizophrenia. Athens: IETHS*. She is a member of the Hellenic Society for Behavioral Research and Therapy (www.eees.gr), of the Bundesverband Deutsche Psychologen und Psychologinnen (BDP) (www.bdp.org), and of the American Psychological Association (www.apa.org), srakitzi@gmail.com, https://www.linkedin.com/in/stavroula-rakitzi-0b512b45/, https://www.psychologenportal.de//karte/stavroylarakitzi.html, www.researchgate.net, http://orcid.org/0000-0002-5231-6619, Twitter: @SSrakitzi, Web of Science Researcher ID: AAT-7720-2020.

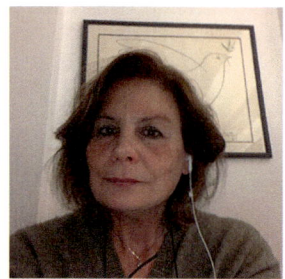

Polyxeni Georgila   is a psychiatrist in private practice and the former director of the adult psychiatry department at the General Hospital "G. Gennimatas" in Athens, Greece. She completed her medicine studies at the University of Athens and specialized in neurology and psychiatry at Eginition Hospital in Athens, Greece. She completed the Professor Papakostas's cognitive therapy program at Eginition Hospital. Not only that, but she was trained in the psychiatric department at the Karolinska Institute in Saint Görans Hospital by Professor Wettenberg. Furthermore, she was a member of the mental health committee of the Greek Ministry of Health. Her clinical and research interests focus on all psychiatric disorders. She co-developed the Integrated Psychological Therapy (IPT) postgraduate program for psychologists and psychiatrists in Greece and trained in CBT.

She has participated in many national and international conferences as a speaker and authored articles in Greek and international journals and books. Furthermore, she is an editor of the Greek book *Intervention in Schizophrenia. Athens: IETHS*. She is a member of the Hellenic Psychiatric Association and the Hellenic Association of Clinical Psychopharmacology. polyxenigeorgila@gmail.com, https://gr.linkedin.com/in/polyxeni-georgila-940b521a7, http://orcid.org/0000-0003-3137-506x

Abbreviations

CBT	Cognitive behavioral therapy
CT-R	Recovery-oriented cognitive therapy
MCT	Metacognitive training
RECOVERYTRSBDGR	Greek recovery-oriented model for TRSBD
TRSBD	Treatment-resistant bipolar disorder

List of Figures

List of Tables

Introduction

Bipolar disorder and treatment-resistant bipolar disorder (TRSBD) display chronic mental health disorders related to high vulnerability, stigma, and suicidality for individuals and their families. So, it is exceptionally vital for us, as mental health experts, to distribute a book centered on bipolar disorder and TRSBD. These disorders merit our consideration, dedication, and willingness to implement research protocols regarding the efficacy and effectiveness of evidence-based interventions and to implement evidence-based interventions by these individuals and finally, they deserve our capability to give the appropriate diagnosis as soon as possible. All these procedures should be done with transparency and polished skill.

Chronic mental disorders, such as bipolar disorders and psychoses or schizophrenia, are characterized by many years of endeavors to stabilize the clinical status after numerous hospitalizations, relapses, suicide, and conflicts within the family! Tolerating the disorders, locking in successful treatments, and moving into recovery take a long time. Things do not alter overnight! Patients and their families ought to be included from the beginning in evidence-based treatments that are actualized on a long-term premise.

Stigma could be a gigantic issue in chronic mental health disorders. Patients and their families put negative labels on themselves as a result of the disorders, and on the other hand, they moreover acknowledge the stigma attached to them by society. This vicious cycle leads to separation, self-destruction, postponing looking for assistance from mental health experts, and overwhelming depression and hopelessness.

The stigma and existence of a chronic mental disorder leads to chronic grief for patients and their families. Grief can lead to segregation and self-destruction if left untreated. The five well-known stages of grief-denial, anger, bargaining, depression, and acceptance—one ought to be involved with the assistance of mental health experts. So it will be less demanding to acknowledge and restart life in a new reasonable setting.

S. Rakitzi, P. Georgila, *Treatment-Resistant Bipolar Disorder*, https://doi.org/10.1007/978-3-031-59001-6_1

TRSBD presents a chronic mental health disorder. An unremitting mental health disorder implies chronic psychiatric treatment in combination with a long-term psychotherapy and rehabilitation. Is this circumstance simple? Of course not! Patients with TRSBD and their families ought to learn to convert this long-term troublesome circumstance into a challenging situation in which they are the heroes in their possess lives which means that they are responsible for more cooperation centered on step-by-step mindfulness and advancement. Evidence-based recovery-oriented treatments contribute to that direction.

What is really a TRSBD? A disorder in which particular agents and a combination of them are effective for these patients. Pharmacotherapy ought to be combined with long-term recovery-oriented psychotherapy and rehabilitation. This is often fundamental since TRSBD is related with high suicidal risk, poor adherence to treatments, cognitive dysfunctions, and hopelessness for their condition. So, it is exceptionally imperative for mental health experts to be taught in an appropriate way, so that they can express empathy toward patients with TRSBD and their families.

Clinical psychiatrists, clinical psychologists, and cognitive behavioral psychotherapists require suitable training, as portrayed by psychiatric associations, psychological associations, and cognitive behavioral associations all over the world. Long-term training is always appropriate in order to be informed and trained in evidence-based interventions.

Psychiatric conferences all over the world incorporate continuous symposia around TRSBD, displaying upgrades with respect to the viability of evidence-based interventions in TRSBD and complications within the treatment. High suicidality could be a gigantic issue in TRSBD, and therefore it is critical to grant the appropriate diagnosis as soon as possible. Our involvement with these people includes numerous cases of people who were undiscovered or who have been given the diagnosis after numerous hospitalizations. Moreover, people with TRSBD are often victims of malpractice from mental health experts who select polypharmacy with dangerous side effects or non-evidence-based interventions in psychotherapy.

Patients with TRSBD merit our capability to battle against malpractice among mental health experts, to give them a straightforward and democratic context to be treated as human beings, who can be dynamic individuals in our society finding a new meaning in life.

This book centers on the clinical components of TRSBD, such as diagnostic procedures, epidemiology, and comorbidity. The current evidence-based interventions for TRSBD in pharmacotherapy, cognitive behavioral psychotherapy, and rehabilitation will be talked about. A new recovery-oriented model centered on the combination of evidence-based pharmacotherapy and psychotherapy will be displayed and examined.

The book is the result of long-term clinical experience and effective cooperation between the two authors in Greece all these years. Clinical psychiatrists and clinical psychologists, who offer cognitive behavioral psychotherapy and rehabilitation to people with bipolar disorder and TRSBD, should cooperate with each other under the conditions of common coexistence and interaction in favor of people with TRSBD.

Long-term evidence-based pharmacotherapy and psychotherapy lead to the transformation of patients with bipolar disorder and TRSBD from inactive, on-edge, suspicious, and frail people to dynamic, mindful, responsible, and more optimistic individuals in a long-term dynamic changing process, step by step, which lead to a better reintegration into society. As a result of this, those people are active members of our society, who attempt to be as assertive as possible regarding their own life goals and their human rights in society.

The protagonists of this book are the individuals who suffer from bipolar disorder and TRSBD and their own families. In this manner, this book is composed in such a way that it can be read easily not only by experts but also by non-experts, such as the above- mentioned protagonists. Additionally, our work aims to protect these people from malpractice and abusive interventions in pharmacotherapy and psychotherapy. They can have a clear picture of what implies evidence-based interventions in mental health. A diagnosis of a chronic mental health disorder presents a difficult context. It is a kind of trauma. Additionally, when non-evidence-based interventions are implemented, a second trauma is created, which has negative long-term consequences such as stigma, social isolation, pessimism, and no adherence to the therapy. People lose their own trust in clinical psychiatrists and clinical psychologists.

Nowadays, the evidence-based interventions in pharmacotherapy and psychotherapy for TRSBD, prove that there is always a right path and setting in which issues can be dealt with. That's the finest reply to malpractice, and thus the authors would like to send a central message through this book: trust evidence-based interventions, no matter how troublesome the circumstance is.

More research studies with respect to the efficacy of evidence-based pharmacotherapy and psychotherapies for TRSBD are requested. Meta-analyses, randomized controlled trials, and other sorts of studies with respect to the efficacy of interventions by patients with TRSBD ought to continuously clarify whether the treatments are efficacious for TRSBD.

It could be a human right to endure from a mental health disorder, such a unremitting mental health disorder as bipolar disorder and TRSBD; it could be a human right to be defenseless and frail and to have get to evidence-based treatments for the most excellent conceivable reintegration into society.

Mental health experts who do not regard the essential human rights of patients with constant mental health disorders ought to be avoided and be beneath the assessment of the ethical committees of the psychiatric and psychological associations.

The European Union and other nations must ensure vulnerable people with mental health disorders through a universal hotline and a group of researchers who will assess whether mental health experts have applied dangerous treatments to TRSBD and appeared to have committed professional misconduct.

This will be a genuine democratic context in which experts and researchers are assessed throughout their entirety professional careers. Experts have the power to help and to contribute to a reintegration into society but they too have the power to devastate the lives of patients with TRSBD, in case they do not follow the ethical standards of the treatments.

Nowadays we cannot accept that evidence-based interventions with respect to pharmacotherapy and psychotherapy for patients with TRSBD are not accessible to the scientific community and to patients with TRSBD and their families.

Scientific associations offer training regarding these interventions within the setting of long-term education. Participation in these trainings must be an obligation to stay updated and to offer sufferers the most excellent conceivable reintegration into society. A long-term education of experts ensures the patients with TRSBD and their families.

Pharmacotherapy is the main therapy for patients with treatment-resistant bipolar disorder. It takes time to give the appropriate diagnosis and to prescribe the right combination of medication. A monthly psychiatric treatment should evaluate all the risks and protective factors. Compliance with pharmacotherapy is always a problem for those patients. So it is very crucial to find as soon as possible the best combination of agents with as few as possible side effects.

A new recovery-oriented program for TRSBD will be displayed. A combination of evidence-based interventions is at the cutting edge.

This model is the result of a long-term clinical encounter and the cooperation of the two authors. It includes three points of view: the cognitive perspective-thoughts and beliefs about problems and incapacity; the metacognitive perspective-thoughts about thoughts and convictions and the recovery perspective-mental health experts, and patients with TRSBD and their families evaluate during the whole life the impact of the evidence-based interventions throughout their lives. This cohesive context helps mental health experts and patients with TRSBD to work together in a dynamic and long-term process that gives individuals meaning in their lives.

Inability and issues with functional outcomes will be treated step by step, dynamic, problem-solving-oriented, long-term, and in a democratic context, in which its conclusion is critical.

Our recovery-oriented model presents a modern option in modern mental health treatment. TRSBD is related with numerous disappointed moments, and patients with TRSBD discontinue exceptionally regularly their therapy. Our recovery-oriented model offers a setting that gives the plausibility for a long-term treatment and a secure therapeutic relationship.

Our long-term clinical involvement with TRSBD led to the disclosure of a modern recovery-oriented model. Dissatisfaction, numerous backslides, high suicidal risk, and numerous treatments without any participation between them are some of the problems of patients with TRSBD. In this manner, our recovery-oriented model tries to offer a long-term cohesive setting for tending to all the issues of TRSBD in a steady therapeutic context.

Patients with TRSBD can feel secure and see modern measurements and outcomes in their lives when they have the chance to get it their issue with straightforwardness and trustworthiness, and mental health experts clarify to them how the issues are communicated, how they can be adapted and how vital it is to be the protagonist of your own problems. Our recovery-oriented therapy takes after the above attitude and structure.

Our recovery-oriented model was born in Athens, Greece. Greece has been gone up against with a socio-economic crisis from 2008 until nowadays. So, this crisis and the different issues of our patients with TRSBD and their families have propelled us to create such a program in a nation such as Greece, which doesn't have contributed enough funds in research in mental health disorders and doesn't invest also enough funds for the public mental health services.

It is exceptionally vital to offer to vulnerable patients new opportunities with respect to psychotherapy and rehabilitation. A socio-economic crisis ought to continuously be a chance to make a defensive setting for patients with chronic mental health disorders and their families. This means that resilience presents the leading arrangement after a social crisis.

Our commitment to the scientific community is to offer the best possible interventions for patients with TRSBD and their families. Sharing and giving the best possible solutions to long-lasting mental health problems, such as TRSBD, is one of the most challenging moments for us.

The contribution of mental health experts to the scientific community is the combination of clinical and research work. The research protocols show us which interventions are compelling, where there are issues with each treatment, and what must be made strides within the future.

We are responsible to patients with persistent mental health disorders and must offer evidence-based interventions. We are obliged to secure them from interventions that are not viable and to clarify to them what is viable for their issue and what isn't. In this way, patients with TRSBD must be treated slightest once a month by a clinical psychiatrist and take part in cognitive-behavioral psychotherapy and rehabilitation programs amid their lives.

The implementation of non-evidence-based psychiatric and psychotherapeutic treatments isn't predicted by any scientific association nowadays. The research data on the adequacy and viability of treatments for TRSBD are indisputable. In this way, the implementation of non-evidence- based interventions is an abuse of power on the portion of mental health experts.

Evidence-based interventions meet the following criteria: they have a specific goal or objectives; they have a manual that gives enlightening on how the treatment can be actualized; and there are studies and meta-analysis with respect to their effectiveness and efficacy.

The therapeutic relationship with patients with TRSBD has limits and objectives. Any violation of these boundaries, such as building up a personal relationship with patients, is additionally an abuse of power. The therapeutic relationship with patients with TRSBD may be a long-term relationship in which patients must believe and incline on therapists to initiate small and expansive changes in their lives.

Hence, mental health experts are called upon to reply to this relationship by appearing the limits and objectives of this relationship.

Our recovery-oriented model shows how a therapeutic relationship with boundaries and goals can be built, through which evidence-based interventions can be executed. Finally, our model protects patients TRSBD and their families from abusive behaviors and abuse of power.

Our recovery-oriented model contributes to the improvement of functional outcomes and the awareness of the disorder that can be expanded. This reduces stigma, which is the worst enemy of people with chronic mental disorders and TRSBD. Stigma presents a forceful behavior that leads to social separation and the avoidance of treatments.

At last, our recovery-oriented model shows a structured way to bargain with fundamental issues in TRSBD. It gives trust and a plausibility to restart life after repeated failed treatment endeavors with TRSBD.

Bipolar disorder can be portrayed as a sea, which changes concurring to weather conditions. When the disposition is sweet and the individual is in great spirits, at that point we see a calm and clean sea, which welcomes us to go and bathe. When the disposition is depressive or the individual is in a hypo manic or manic state, and after that the sea is stormy, dirty and unsafe. He warns us not to go inside and see her from a far distance. We'll got to hold up for it to calm down.

Our recovery-oriented model leads to more resilience; it reinforces positive beliefs about life and what an individual can do. Thus knowing on the one hand the vulnerabilities and shortcomings and on the other the positive things that one can accomplish, one chooses reasonable objectives with more resilience and optimism.

Building resilience creates citizens who can claim their rights within a democratic society. A democratic society and scientists must provide the appropriate tools, such as effective treatments, so that our frail fellow citizens, such as those with chronic mental disorders, can reintegrate into society with realistic possibilities. Let us all join forces in this direction.

The execution of an effective therapeutic program must center on addressing the fundamental issues of chronic mental disorder and on the other hand respond to the high ideals of a democratic society, which must support our vulnerable fellow citizens in their reintegration into society. The creation of our program has been a very beautiful journey for us taking into account our knowledge and clinical experience, the requirements of patients with TRSBD and their families, modern and evidence-based treatments and the avoidance of abusive practices in clinical practice.

Structured and effective evidence-based psychotherapy leads to a new way of considering and dealing with circumstances, regulation of daily life, and accomplishing new objectives. This learning process is stored within in the memory of the individual and is slowly connected consequently to regular life. Hence, there are frequently back slides and surprises because this mechanism is activated and sets a limit on the impulsive and juvenile way of thinking and action.

This self-regulation mechanism is in other words an awfully good filter before one acts, which assesses the data and determines a sensible way of reaction. In other words, this mechanism maybe a life compass! This reliefs and leads to new perspectives in life. So the past with many traumas, disappointments in treatments and relapses no longer guides the present. This is directly influenced by this psychotherapeutic mechanism of self-regulation.

Recovery-oriented psychotherapy is in this manner not as it were approximately reducing symptoms and improving quality of life and functional outcome. Psychotherapy is an add up to restart of life with new principles, values, realistic expectations, and a positive orientation in life.

The protection of human rights and freedoms is not something hypothetical and philosophical. It ought to take shape in numerous areas through different actions. Thus, mental health ought to be ensured by the application of effective and evidence-based treatments, which increment the plausibility of reintegration into society in the best conceivable conditions.

In case of mental health professionals to implement effective and evidence-based treatments, at that point we superior to protect the human rights and freedoms of our patients and their families.

Especially in resistant forms of mental health disorders, such as TRSBD, the protection of the human rights and freedoms of patients gets to be indeed more vital. Patients with TRSBD regularly involvement experience relapses and frequently alters mental health professionals. They lose their trust and confidence in science. So our responsibility is incredible toward this category of people.

Thus, the usage of an evidence-based therapy is not only aimed at solving problems so that reintegration into society is conceivable, but also at the sacred good of ensuring human rights. In other words, the role of the mental health experts also focuses on securing the value and dignity of human life beneath any troublesome condition.

Protecting the value and dignity of human life is a supreme good and goal for all of us scientists. This ought to be our ultimate goal.

In case we don't accomplish this goal at that point, then any effectiveness or viability of a treatment is of no value. Effectiveness must be communicated in down to earth results in important areas of our lives, driving to more dignity and protection of human life.

Patients with chronic mental health disorders, and particularly with TRSBD, are frequently incapable to protect their lives, the dignity of their lives and their security. The combination of evidence-based pharmacotherapy and psychotherapy has as a common objective that the individual learns to protect himself and the dignity of his life.

The target groups in the book are medicine and psychology students, scientists, and researchers in psychology and psychiatry, clinical psychologists, and clinical psychiatrists, cognitive behavioral psychotherapists and psychotherapists, and, at long last, people who suffer from TRSBD and their families.

Competing Interests The authors have no conflicts of interest to declare that are pertinent to the content of this chapter.

Recovery in Chronic Mental Health Disorders, Especially in Bipolar Disorder, and in Treatment-Resistant Bipolar Disorder

2

Learning Objects

1. The therapeutic relationship for the recovery process in chronic mental health disorders.
2. How can we form an effective relationship with patients with TRSBD?
3. Definition of recovery.
4. The recovery process in bipolar disorder and TRSBD.

2.1   The Recovery Process and Its Significance

Chronic mental health disorders are associated with emotional burden across the lifespan and with high vulnerability. The diagnosis of a chronic mental health disorder, such as bipolar disorder, is made early in life, when patients are young. Such a diagnosis prevents solid advancement and a feasible future.

The earlier evidence-based pharmacotherapy and psychotherapy starts, the better it is for the patients and their families. Recovery-oriented treatment proactively addresses issues associated with chronic mental health disorders, slowing disease progression and helping to prevent the emergence of complex comorbidities. These circumstances increment the probability of a more secure and relentless future in the setting of chronic mental health disorders.

Professionals, such as clinical psychiatrists, clinical psychologists, and cognitive-behavioral psychotherapists, strive to build stable, safe, long-term therapeutic relationships with patients with chronic mental disorders, such as TRSBD, who are in the recovery process. A long-term therapeutic relationship means a long-term commitment of the professionals to the treatment, long-term supervision as well as peer supervision of the professionals in the treatment of chronic mental health disorders, and finally, proper psycho-hygiene of the experts so they can relax and take care of themselves. This procedure activates resources and motivates the specialist to

© The Author(s), under exclusive license to Springer Nature
Switzerland AG 2024
S. Rakitzi, P. Georgila, *Treatment-Resistant Bipolar Disorder*,
https://doi.org/10.1007/978-3-031-59001-6_2

continue long-term treatment. Professionals should motivate patients with TRSBD in every session to achieve a better quality of life and fight for their reintegration into society.

Empathy, acceptance, and positive communication are key characteristics needed to build a good long-term therapeutic relationship in the context of psychiatric treatment, cognitive behavioral therapy, and rehabilitation. The therapeutic alliance is an important part of the therapeutic relationship and contributes to therapeutic boundaries (respect, trust, and appreciation). Four key elements are important to improve the therapeutic relationship and alliance: guided discovery through Socratic questioning, consulting skills, collaborative empiricism, and case formulation [1]. A good long-term therapeutic relationship with TRSBD must be combined with the use of specific pharmacological and CBT interventions so that improvements can be achieved at multiple levels. A modern evidence-based intervention must make recovery the ultimate objective of all treatments. Recovery should be assessed before, after treatment, and at follow-up a few months later. In other words, recovery must be archived.

There are two definitions of recovery: recovery as an outcome (objective recovery), which presents the opinions of experts and is assessed by psychometric tests. Recovery as a process (subjective recovery) represents the perspective of people with mental health disorders and their families. This opinion emphasizes the fact that the recovery process and its evaluation are dynamic and continuous. Both perspectives are vital and must be considered [2].

There are numerous psychometric tests assessing treatment outcomes in bipolar disorder and TRSBD, such as the Symptoms Rating Scale for Depression and Anxiety (SRSDSA) [3, 4], the Altman Self-Rating Mania Scale [5], SCL-90-R for depression [6], the psychotic symptom rating scales (PSYRATS) [7], WHODAS 2 0 [8, 9] for disability and functional outcomes, and the Recovery Domains and Stages Assessment Scale (RAS-DS), which presents a valid and reliable tool for assessing recovery [10–14]. RAS-DS presents a self-report outcome measure that is translated into 18 languages. The following areas are evaluated: doing things I care about, looking forward to the future, managing my illness, connecting, and belonging [10, 13, 14]. RAS-DS is translated in Greek by Dr. Rakitzi and Mrs. Sofia Katoudi (Msc). RAS-DS is used systematically by Dr. Rakitzi to evaluate the adequacy of psychotherapy, and it will also be utilized for the assessment of the effectiveness and efficacy of RECOVERYTRSGR, as depicted in Chap. 4 of this book. RAS-DS is a really curiously scale since it measures all the components of recovery and all these things that can donate meaning to life. It is not only the functional outcome that is important for the outcome of psychotherapy. Recovery is also crucial as an outcome, especially when it is assessed as a self-report.

It is specifically to evaluate recovery in TRSBD. Recovery in depression implies that there is a balance every day toward depressive temperament so that the individual can reach the recovery goals in RAS-DS and recovery in hypo-manic or manic mood implies to that individuals found a balance to decrease hypo-mania or mania and to reach recovery goals.

TRSBD is a chronic mental health disorder, meaning recovery is a dynamic process that keeps going all through life. Individuals with TRSBD start with long-term recovery-oriented pharmacotherapy and psychotherapy.

Evidence-based pharmacotherapy is centered on the choice of the suitable agents or the combination of them to achieve remission and recovery without unsafe side effects.

Recovery as an outcome (objective recovery) implies that clinical psychiatrists ought to evaluate the result of the pharmacotherapy before and after 3, 6, 12, 24, etc., months from the starting of the treatment.

Evidence-based psychotherapy is a vital complement to pharmacotherapy.

Psycho-education is the primary step, helping people better understand and become more aware of this disorder. Cognitive-behavioral psychotherapy and rehabilitation improve symptoms, cognitive functioning, and functional outcomes, promoting social reintegration at multiple levels. All of these interventions contribute to remission. Individuals with TRSBD should receive training in relapse prevention, so they can recognize any early signs of relapse. Eventually, recovery will be the outcome and will be assessed. This procedure is never-ending in the context of chronic mental health disorders. Patients with TRSBD and their families work alongside mental health professionals.

Recovery as an outcome demonstrates the obligation of professionals to patients with TRSBD and their families. They are dependable in giving evidence-based treatments and assessing their effectiveness and efficiency.

Recovery as a process involves the obligation of patients with TRSBD and their families to receive treatment. They ought to take as long as necessary to get forward their symptoms and vulnerabilities; they ought to consult experts if they have trouble integrating treatments into their daily routine; and they ought to stand up for more rights in society beneath the authority of experts.

In other words, patients with TRSBD are protagonists, and this dynamic role in their own problems strengthens their resilience. Evidence-based treatment of TRSBD begins with evidence-based, recovery-oriented treatments and continues with recovery (outcomes and processes) all through life expectancy. This procedure gives people new meaning in their lives!

The recovery perspective (recovery as an outcome and recovery as a process) offers numerous focal points. It is a democratic context in which mental health experts, patients with TRSBD, and their families, talk straightforwardly approximately the positive and negative results of treatments and how the negative results can be changed. It is additionally a dynamic process that goes on and gives the opportunity to be assessed within the long term. This process gives patients a modern meaning in their lives and mental health experts more openings to extend the plausibility of victory by executing interventions. In other words, the recovery perspective battles against narcissism, arrogance, cynicism, and the indifference of the mental health experts. The recovery perspective shows the real democracy and collaboration.

The recovery perspective focuses on change, activation of resources, self- responsibility, hope, and on including new dimensions in their possess lives. It isn't sufficient to acknowledge a troublesome and chronic mental health disorder and to learn to live with it in accordance. It is essential to alter and progress the disabilities step by step, in an organized and practical way, and to set the objective of focusing on long-term alter and upgrade.

Mental health experts ought to be prepared for recovery-oriented treatments. It isn't sufficient to accept a difficult mental health disorder, such as TRSBD. It is vital to bring about changes that lead to a new restart in life concurring to the life circumstances. This issue will be realized through recovery-oriented interventions. Alter and transformation are the most vital conditions for recovering from a chronic mental health condition.

The efficacy of evidence-based interventions in TRSBD in various settings, such as ambulant settings, hospitals, day centers, etc., ought to be assessed from a recovery perspective. Which levels of recovery has the patient of TRSBD accomplished, and how can this demonstrate through recovery as an outcome and recovery as a process? Each mental health expert should be obliged to execute recovery-oriented interventions that lead to reintegration into society in a straightforward and effective way.

Mental health experts have the power to alter the lives of patients with TRSBD and their families. In the case, this power is misused, the results are catastrophic for the patients. A recovery-oriented point of view and therapy displays a channel between mental health experts and patients with TRSBD, which secures patients from misconduct and misuse. Mental health experts should be under long-lasting evaluation from the patients with TRSBD and their families. Patients ought to be assertive about every violation of their rights and each execution of non-evidence-based interventions.

TRSBD is like an enormous journey in numerous ways. Some of them are easy to do; others are troublesome and require consideration and adaptability. Patients with TRSBD learn to coexist with their disorder peacefully in way without shame, stigma, or guilt. They have the right to be vulnerable and to adapt their reality to the new conditions. It is imperative that patients remain alone all through their lives, under the direction of mental health professionals. These strategies give people new meaning in their possessed lives!

Recovery is a critical point of view that we had to incorporate. It will lead to changes and new adaptations in life. It isn't enough to acknowledge the problem and learn to oversee it. We need to train the people in the recovery perspective to implement the appropriate changes as soon as possible.

Taken together, the recovery perspective and its importance were talked about, Recovery was defined, and psychometric tests that assess recovery were displayed. Finally, the advantages of the recovery process were also discussed.

2.2   Conclusions

Long-term therapeutic relationships between mental health professionals and patients with TRSBD in recovery are appropriate so that they can feel safe and stable to continue their recovery process. The recovery as an outcome and the recovery as a process represent two perspectives equally important to TRSBD.

Revision Questions
1. Why is it important to build a good therapeutic relationship in the context of the recovery of chronic mental health disorders?
2. Which factors contribute to a therapeutically positive change in TRSBD?
3. Define recovery.
4. Describe the recovery process in TRSBD.

Competing Interests   The authors have no conflicts of interest to declare that are relevant to the content of this chapter.

References

1. Kazantzis N, Dattilio FM, Dobson KS. The therapeutic relationship in cognitive-behavioral therapy: a clinician's guide. New York: Guilford Publication; 2017.
2. Leonhardt BL, Huling K, Hamm JA, Roe D, Hasson-Ohayon I, McLeod HM, et al. Recovery and serious mental illness: a review of current and clinical and research paradigms and future directions. Exp Rev Neurotherapeut. 2017;17:1117–30. https://doi.org/10.1080/14737175.2017.1378099.
3. Bech P. Rating scales for psychopathology, health status and quality of life. Berlin: Springer; 1993. p. 325–40.
4. Fountoulakis KN, Iacovides A, Kleanthous S, Samolis S, Gougoulias K, Kaprinis G, Bech P. The Greek translation of the symptoms rating scale for depression and anxiety: preliminary results of the validation study. BMC Psychiatry. 2003;3:21. http://www.biomedcentral.com/1471-244X/3/21.
5. Altman EG, Hedecker D, Peterson JL, Davis M. The Altman self-rating mania scale. Soc Biol Psychiat. 1997;42:948–55.
6. Donias S, Karastergiou A, Manos N. Standardization of the symptom checklist-90-R rating scale in a Greek population. Psychiatrist. 1991;2(1):42–8.
7. Haddock G, McCarron J, Tarrier N, Faragher EB. Scales to measure dimensions of hallucinations and delusions: the psychotic symptom rating scales (PSYRATS). Psychol Med. 1999;29(4):879–89.
8. World Health Organization. International classification of functioning, disability and health (ICF). Geneva: World Health Organization; 2001.
9. Koumpouros Y, Papageorgiou E, Sakellari E, et al. Adaptation and psychometric properties' evaluation of the Greek version of WHODAS 2.0. Pilot application in Greek elderly population. Health Serv Outcome Res Methodol. 2018;18(1):63–74. https://doi.org/10.1007/s10742-017-0176-x.
10. Hancock N, Scanlan JN, Bundy AC, Honey A. Recovery assessment scale –domains & stages (RAS-DS) manual-version 3. Sydney: University of Sydney; 2019.

11. Hancock N, Rakitzi S, Katoudi S. Recovery assessment scale-domains & stages (RAS-DS). The Greek version; 2023.
12. Hancock N, Scanlan J, Honey A, Bundy A, O'Shea K. Recovery assessment scale – domains & stages (RAS-DS): its feasibility and outcome measurement capacity. Austr New Zeal J Psychiatry. 2015;49(7):624633. https://doi.org/10.1177/0004867414564084.
13. Ramesh S, Scanlan JN, Honey A, Hancock N. Feasibility of recovery assessment scale-domains and stages (RAS-DS) for every day mental health practice. Front Psych. 2024;15:1256092. https://doi.org/10.3389/fpsyt.2024.1256092.
14. Honey A, Hancock N, Scanlan JN. Staff perceptions of factors affecting the use of RAS-DS to support collaborative mental health practice. BMC Psychiatry. 2023;23:500. https://doi.org/10.1186/s12888-023-04996-2.

Treatment-Resistant Bipolar Disorder

3

Learning Objectives
1. Definition of bipolar disorder
2. Definition of TRSBD.
3. Why is TRSBD difficult?
4. Evidence-based pharmacotherapy for TRSBD.
5. Evidence-based psychotherapy for TRSBD.

3.1 Introduction

Bipolar disorder, and especially treatment-resistant bipolar disorder (TRSBD), presents a chronic mental health disorder that influences the quality of life and the functional outcome of patients with TRSBD and their families. The sooner a substantial diagnosis is given, the better for the individual and their family.

International scientific associations recommend guidelines regarding the evidence-based pharmacotherapy and psychotherapy of bipolar disorder and TRSBD [1, 2]. These rules ought to be taken carefully into consideration.

There are three elements that are suitable to arrange to provide the definition of treatment resistance in mental health disorders: the right diagnosis has been given, the suitable treatment has been offered, but there is an inadequate response to the therapy. Treatment resistance is categorized as primary (early onset) at the early beginning of pharmacotherapy and secondary (late onset) a good response at the beginning is followed by an inadequate response to treatment over time [3].

TRSBD is characterized as a disappointment to attain symptomatic reduction for 8 weeks after two diverse medicines at satisfactory restorative dosages with at least two monotherapy medicines or at very least one monotherapy [4].

Patients with bipolar disorder, especially Bipolar I and II disorders, appear to have neurocognitive dysfunctions. Bipolar I disorder appears to have a higher

© The Author(s), under exclusive license to Springer Nature
Switzerland AG 2024
S. Rakitzi, P. Georgila, *Treatment-Resistant Bipolar Disorder*,
https://doi.org/10.1007/978-3-031-59001-6_3

burden with respect to cognitive dysfunction [5]. Individuals with bipolar disorder show psychomotor retardation and impaired memory in comparison to healthy individuals. Individuals in the manic phase show bigger impairments in verbal memory, visual memory and executive functioning in comparison to hypomanic, depressive, and euthymic bipolar patients [6].

Considering the above empirical data, TRSBD needs more time for the choice of the appropriate pharmacotherapy. This is associated with cognitive deficits, which have a negative impact on daily routine and quality of life. The sooner the diagnosis is given, the better the choice of appropriate pharmacotherapy. After the stabilization of the individuals with TRSBD, regarding pharmacotherapy, the implementation of evidence-based psychotherapies follows. When the above strategy isn't followed, the risk of dismal hospitalizations and self-destructive behavior is exceptionally high.

This procedure contributes to the confidence in evidence-based interventions.

Polypharmacy presents a phenomenon to which individuals with TRSBD are stood up. It is related to unsafe side effects that lead to the individual passing away or to exceptionally awful adherence to agents and a dropout from the pharmacotherapy.

Non-evidence-based psychotherapies lead exceptionally dangerous results because they are not structured and goal oriented. The main psychotherapeutic objectives are the decrease of depressive and manic-hypomanic symptoms, the improvement of cognitive functions, and the upgrade of quality of life and functional outcome under the recovery perspective. Those therapeutic goals are taken care of evidence-based psychotherapies.

Electroconvulsive Therapy (ECT) is compelling in bipolar depression. It is recommended after three fizzled trials with pharmacotherapy or as a last step when most biological treatment didn't succeed. The most common sign for ECT is depression, followed by (psychotic) mania. ECT is exceptionally compelling for all bipolar acute depressive, mixed, and manic episodes that do not respond to routine pharmacotherapy. It got to be considered as a treatment of choice in patients with extraordinary depressive and mixed states with delirious and catatonic features. Further research with respect to the efficacy of ECT and the effect on cognitive function is required [7–10].

Nowadays, ECT ought be the final arrangement in exceptionally emotional cases of TRSBD because it has already been pointed out. Our priority in TRSBD is to continue the appropriate pharmacotherapy in secure doses combined with long-term evidence-based psychotherapy.

Working with chronic mental health disorders, such as TRSBD could be an extraordinary challenge. The long-term collaboration with the patients and their families driven us to restructure our own beliefs as mental health experts toward bipolar disorder and TRSBD.

Patience, structured-oriented techniques, motivation-oriented and recovery-oriented therapeutic skills are critical to managing conceivable frustration during the long-term therapeutic process.

Additionally, mental health experts ought to look out themselves and discover time during the week to relax, to spend time with family and companions, and to prepare themselves for the next week with all these restorative sessions with sufferers of TRSBD. A long-term treatment for TRSBD implies more prominent duty and cohesion, as well as step-by-step recovery on all imperative levels, such as cognitive, emotional, and behavioral levels, functional outcome and quality of life.

The therapeutic relationship with TRSBD has two phases: The primary phase is the getting-to-know-you phase, recording what has not gone well so far as well as the advantages and disadvantages of previous interventions. In this way, mental health experts are listeners and provide a platform to express the negative contemplations and sentiments of patients with TRSBD and their families.

Empathy toward the issues of the past is the fundamental principle and strategy. The second part of the relationship goes into activity and intervention by straightforwardly highlighting how the treatment will be done.

Patients with TRSBD and their families are our near accomplices, without whom the treatment cannot be actualized. Intervening in the family and working with them is an exceptionally important portion of the treatment and the therapeutic relationship. In Greece in particular, the majority of TRSBD patients live with their families and have their financial and emotional support.

A democratic society has a responsibility to ensure the human rights of all individuals with mental health disorders and must give rise to evidence-based pharmacotherapy and psychotherapy.

Taken together, bipolar disorder and TRSBD display chronic mental health disorders with consequences for quality of life and functional outcomes. The sooner a diagnosis is given, the better for the patients. Long-term evidence-based pharmacotherapy and psychotherapy should be the first choice. Polypharmacy and non-evidence-based psychotherapies should be avoided. ECT should be chosen under specific circumstances. Working with mental health disorders presents a great responsibility for mental health experts. Experts are obliged to protect the human rights of patients with TRSBD.

3.2   Diagnostic Procedure

According to the DSM-5-TR [11], *bipolar I disorder* is characterized by manic, hypomanic, and major depressive episodes. A manic episode contains grandiosity, decreased need for sleep, thoughts racing, distractibility, increased goal-oriented activity, and involvement in activities with negative consequences.

The functional outcome is disturbed. A manic episode leads to hospitalization. A hypomanic episode has the above symptoms but is less severe, needs most of the time no hospitalization, and the functional outcome is not disturbed. If psychotic symptoms arise, then we speak of a manic episode. A major depressive episode has the following symptoms: depressed mood most of the day, decreased interest in many activities, weight loss or gain, insomnia or hypersomnia, psychomotor agitation, loss of energy, excessive guilt, decreased ability to think or concentrate, and suicidal thoughts.

The functional outcome is disturbed. *Bipolar II disorder* contains hypomanic episodes and major depressive episodes, and functional outcome are impaired. *Cyclothymic disorder* is characterized by periods with hypomanic and depressive symptoms that they do not meet criteria for a depressive or a hypomanic episode for at least 2 years.

The symptoms are not explained by another mental health disorder or a medical condition. The disorder causes big problems with functional outcomes [11]. Cyclothymic disorder presents a neurodevelopmental disorder with emotion dysregulation and rapid mood changes at the forefront. 30–50% of individuals with anxiety, depressive disorders, borderline personality disorder, and other personality disorders show cyclothymic disorder [12].

A *differential diagnosis of bipolar I disorder* ought to be made from major depressive disorder, other bipolar disorders, anxiety disorders, substance or medication-induced bipolar disorder, attention/deficit-hyperactive disorder, and personality disorders, such as borderline personality disorder [11].

A *differential diagnosis of bipolar II disorder* ought to be made from major depressive disorder, cyclothymic disorder, schizophrenia and psychotic disorders, anxiety disorders, substance use disorders, from attention/deficit-hyperactive disorder, personality disorders, such as borderline personality disorder, and other bipolar disorders [11].

A differential diagnosis of cyclothymic disorder ought to be made from bipolar and depressive disorder due to a medical condition, from substance-induced bipolar or depressive disorder, from bipolar I and II with rapid cycling, and from borderline personality disorder [11].

Bipolar disorder and TRSBD may coexist with a personality disorder that ought to be diagnosed with DSM-5-TR [11]. Mental health experts ought to center on the treatment of bipolar disorder and TRSBD as a first priority and, secondly, of personality disorders. It can be conceivable that the stabilization of TRSBD can lead to an enhancement in the personality disorder.

The combination of TRSBD and avoidant personality disorder means that the patient feels inferior to others and is very sensitive to rejection and criticism. TRSBD with comorbid dependent personality disorder means that the person cannot live without having dependent relationships in which he/she feels secure and safe and disagreements are not expressed. Obsessive-compulsive personality disorder and TRSBD is characterized by a focus on order, perfectionism, and control.

A narcissistic personality disorder and TRSBD show grandiosity, want to be admired, and has lack of empathy. A histrionic personality disorder and TRSBD seek attention always. A borderline personality disorder and TRSBD show impulsivity, unstable relationships, and suicidal behavior, and feelings of emptiness. TRSBD and antisocial personality disorder violate the rights of others and show criminal behavior. A schizotypal personality disorder and TRSBD shows social and interpersonal deficits, suspiciousness, and magical thinking.

A schizoid personality disorder and TRSBD is isolated from other people, chooses solo activities, takes pleasure in few activities, and has no close friends. A paranoid personality disorder and TRSBD show a lack of trust toward others and suspiciousness.

A dual diagnosis of TRSBD and a serious personality disorder presents an awfully troublesome issue. It is well known that a severe personality disorder makes everything difficult, including the therapeutic relationship. These people have numerous issues building steady relationships with others, showing empathy toward others, and showing respect for the rights of other people. That means that resistant depressive and manic symptoms, cognitive dysfunctions and problems with functional outcomes will be treated more difficultly in combination with a severe personality disorder.

Mixed features of bipolar disorder are present in 40% of the people in this group. They are related to poorer clinical outcomes, greater treatment resistance, higher rates of comorbidity, more frequent mood episodes, and increased rates of suicide [13].

Geriatric bipolar disorder is divided in two groups: people with symptoms, which start earlier in life, and people with late life onset. Medical comorbidity and higher rates of cognitive impairment are the main characteristics of elderly bipolar disorder [14].

There is a moderate support for the idea that unrecognized bipolar disorder contributes to treatment-resistant depression [15].

Traumas display risk factors for the development of severe bipolar disorder [16].

The following psychometric tests are recommended: the semi-structured interview, the schedule for affective disorder and schizophrenia, the General Behavior Inventory, the Mood Disorder Questionnaire, the Bech Rafaelsen Mania Rating Scale, the Altman Self-Rating Mania Scale, and the Self-Rating Mania Inventory to evaluate the symptoms of bipolar disorder [17]. Additionally, the Symptoms Rating Scale for Depression and Anxiety (SRSDSA) [18, 19], SCL-90-R for depression [20], and the psychotic symptom rating scales (PSYRATS) [21] can also be used.

WHODAS 2.0 [22, 23] evaluates the disability and functional outcome, and the Recovery Assessment Scale-Domains and Stages (RAS-DS) [24–26] evaluates the recovery process.

The clinical psychiatrist may recommend in resistant bipolar disorder electroencephalogram, axial or magnetic brain.

Other related disorders that belong to the same category, are substance-medication- induced bipolar and related disorders, bipolar and related disorders due to another medical condition, specified bipolar and related disorders, and unspecified bipolar and related disorders [11]. This book centers on treatment-resistant bipolar I, bipolar II, and cyclothymic disorder.

In sum, there are specific diagnostic criteria for Bipolar I, II disorder and cyclothymic disorder. Psychometric tests can also be implemented. A differential diagnosis should be done carefully. The coexistence of TRSBD and personality disorder should be taken into consideration. 40% of the patients show mixed features.

Geriatric bipolar disorder presents a specific category. Treatment-resistant depression can be associated with unrecognized bipolar disorder. Finally, trauma can be a risk factor for the development of bipolar disorder.

3.3   Epidemiology

The 12-month prevalence of *bipolar I disorder* in the USA is 0.6%. 18 years old is the average age at the onset of *bipolar I disorder.* The 12-month prevalence of *bipolar II disorder* is 0.3% internationally and 0.8% in the USA. The mid-20s are the average age at onset of *bipolar II disorder.* The lifetime prevalence of *cyclothymic disorder* is 0.4–1%, and it ordinarily starts in youth or early adult life [11]. Treatment resistance arises in 20–60% of patients with mental health disorders [3].

3.4   Comorbidity

There are many clinical factors that are related to treatment-resistant bipolar disorder, such as sex (female and older), an older age at illness onset, a high percentage of family depression, unemployment, a high percentage of lifetime stressors, medical problems, comorbid anxiety disorders, and a more regular use of benzodiazepines [27].

The lifetime risk of suicide for individuals with *bipolar disorder I* is very high. 30% of these people have many problems with functional outcomes, especially in their work roles. Suicidal behavior is also very frequent in *bipolar II disorder.* The prevalence of lifetime attempted suicide is 32.4% for *bipolar II disorder* and 36.3% for *bipolar I disorder.* 15% of individuals with *bipolar disorder II* have functional dysfunction between episodes, and 20% of them go directly to another mood episode without recovery. Cognitive dysfunctions present a problem for both *bipolar I and bipolar II disorders.* Dysfunctions in attention, verbal learning and memory, executive functions, and social cognition (the theory of mind) arise frequently in bipolar disorders. 40–60% of people with bipolar disorders suffer from cognitive dysfunction [11, 28, 29].

Alcohol, substance abuse, and anxiety disorders present a frequent comorbidity in bipolar disorder [11, 30, 31]. Attention/deficit-hyperactive disorder, impulse control or conduct disorder, and medical disorders, such as metabolic syndrome and migraine are frequent comorbid disorders in *bipolar I disorder.* 14% of individuals with *bipolar II disorder* develop lifetime eating disorders, such as binge-eating disorders [11].

10% of individuals with borderline personality disorder had bipolar I disorder, and another 10% bipolar II disorder. That means that borderline personality disorder coexists with bipolar disorder, and this should be taken into consideration within the setting of differential diagnosis [32].

There is a 15–50% risk in *cyclothymic disorder* to develop bipolar I or bipolar II disorder. Substance-related and sleep disorders present as comorbid disorders in *cyclothymic disorder*. Children with *cyclothymic disorder* frequently have comorbid attention-deficit hyperactivity disorder [11].

Comorbid disorders caused by TRSBD should be assessed rapidly so that an appropriate therapeutic plan can incorporate them. TRSBD encompasses a very high suicidal risk, which should be treated as a first priority.

Co-occurring personality disorders should be evaluated. A therapeutic plan with respect to intervention for personality disorders ought to be realized after the main treatment for TRSBD. In other words, TRSBD is the priority of the therapy.

Taken together, comorbidity in TRSBD ought to be taken into consideration as soon as conceivable. Suicidal risk, substance abuse disorders, anxiety disorders, cognitive dysfunctions, and personality disorders display the main categories of comorbid disorders in bipolar disorders.

3.5 Evidence-Based Pharmacotherapy, Cognitive Behavioral Psychotherapy, and Rehabilitation in Treatment-Resistant Bipolar Disorder

The main therapy for patients with treatment-resistant bipolar disorder (TRSBD) is the *evidence-based* pharmacotherapy [2, 12, 33–36]. The most recent upgrades with respect to pharmacotherapy for treatment-resistant bipolar disorder will be displayed (Fig. 3.1).

The manic episode in bipolar I disorder can be treated with lithium, which has been available since the late nineteenth century as antimanic medication with great efficacy in 70% of cases have great efficacy with lithium. Furthermore, it is the basic mood stabilizer of bipolar disorder. It is suggested alone in bipolar II and combined to other agents in bipolar I, and in treatment-resistant bipolar disorder. Kidney and thyroid dysfunction are side effects of long-term lithium use and should be medically tested. Lithium blood levels should be monitored. The desired level is 0.6–1 mEq/L to have a reduction in manic symptoms.

Lithium levels of 1–1.2 mEq/L lead to side effects such as diarrhea, fatigue, and drowsiness, and levels of 1.5–2 mEq/L lead to tremors, shakiness, impaired concentration, and memory. Lithium levels above 2 mEq/L lead, respectively, to psoriasis alopecia rash and weight gain, and above 2.5 mEq/L to confusion and coma. Pregnancy is a contraindication because of genetic abnormalities that occur.

Valproate (50–100 µg/ml) is an effective mood stabilizer for the disease. This active substance is metabolized in the liver; it requires good liver function, especially in case of other drugs taken that are metabolized in the liver.

Carbamazepine is effective because it helps to reduce agitation, and levels must be maintained at 4 µg/ml to avoid side effects such as agranulocytosis and pancytopenia. The combination with lithium can be effective in cases of resistant bipolar disease.

There are also newer antiepileptic agents, such as topiramate, pregabalin, and lamotrigine, which can only be used effectively as complementary agents and are effective.

Fig. 3.1 The context of
evidence-based
pharmacotherapy and
psychotherapy for TRSBD

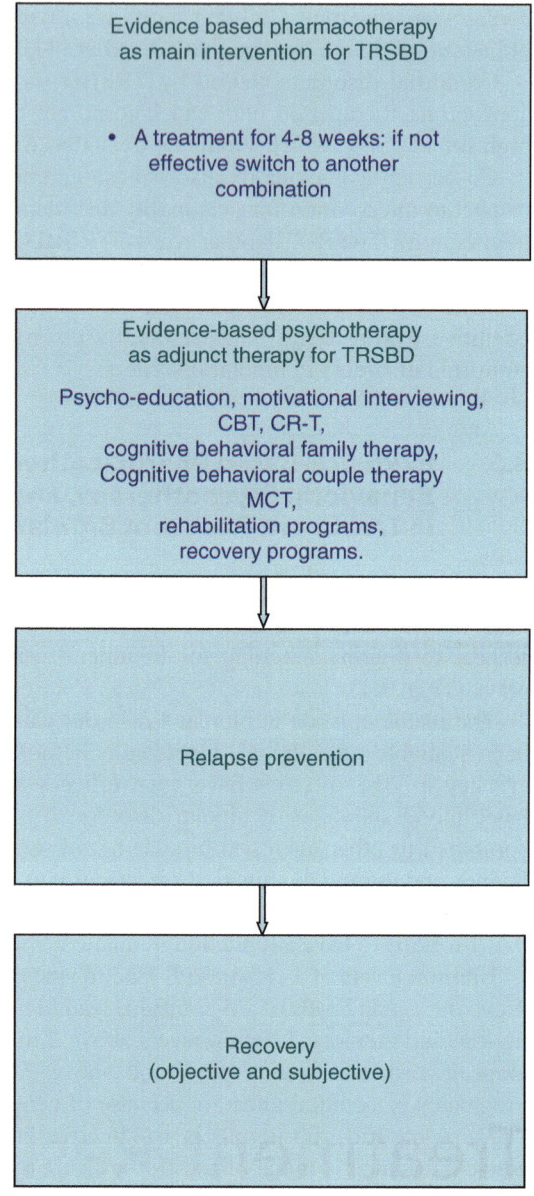

Antipsychotic agents—typical agents (haloperidol, phenothiazines) and atypical agents (clozapine, olanzapine, risperidone, aripiprazole, and quetiapine)—have been used for several years to treat bipolar disorder. The combination of an antipsychotic agent and lithium clearly leads to a more effective response to the manic episodes and undoubtedly the resistant manic episode. At last, the combination of lithium and clozapine is the best possible choice in extreme cases of resistance with all the required follow-up medical tests specifically in the case of clozapine with its known life-threatening side effects, such as accocytaemia, tachycardia torsadis, and heart attack.

Side effects of typical and atypical antipsychotic agents, such as metabolic syndrome, diabetes mellitus, and neuroleptic malignant syndrome, should be always under control. Typical antipsychotic agents are mainly responsible for extrapyramidal dystonia and parkinsonism side effects that have a greater incidence risk in patients with affective disorders than in other psychotic disorders. We may consider it as a useful criterion in the differential diagnosis of bipolar disorder.

Continuous monitoring is necessary because metabolic syndrome can lead to cardiovascular problems, obesity, and poor quality of life as well as poor compliance in the long term. The neuroleptic malignant syndrome is acutely invasive and life-threatening and has a 20% mortality rate.

Antidepressants are divided into specific categories: The administration of antidepressant treatment in bipolar disorder depends on the intensity and duration of the depressive episode. Today, the use of SSRIs is considered as the first-choice treatment (fluoxetine, paroxetine, citalopram, and sertraline). In the case of non-response within 6 weeks, at least two SSRIs are alternated with the final conclusion of the application of an SNRI, such as the venlafaxine and duloxetine. In cases of non-response, there are also older antidepressants, such as the clomipramine and MAO antidepressant agent. Antidepressants such as agomelatine can also be used as alternative. Antidepressant treatment must coexist with a mood stabilizer, with or without an antipsychotic agent.

The dosage of SSRIs can range from 20 to 60 mg, while the SNRIs from 150 to 450 mg in resistant depression. The use of lamotrigine can be used in cases of resistant depression combined to the antidepressive medication.

Lastly, the use of E. C. T (Electroconvulsive therapy) is appropriate in extra resistant cases of depressive episodes, specifically when the patient is in a stupor condition.

The combination of lithium and clozapine is a very good combination for resistant bipolar I disorder with suicidality. But this should be combined with regular psychiatric follow-ups, a very good therapeutic relationship, and an alliance with the family environment. Lithium blood levels should be between 0.6 and 1 mEq/L and clozapine levels over 350 n/ml (100–250 mg).

The use of an antipsychotic agent during life does not always seem to be necessary in bipolar II. On the contrary, the use of an antipsychotic agent stabilizes bipolar I patient's clinical condition in the long term.

In cases of treatment non-compliance in bipolar I, long-acting injectable agents can be used, such as haloperidol (100 mg monthly), olanzapine (300 mg monthly), and aripiprazole (400 mg monthly).

The medical treatment of cyclothymic disorder is a very difficult goal, given the very rapid mood fluctuations and the rules of pharmacodynamics. My clinical experience suggests two or more times a month of follow-up, CBT, and systematic collaboration with the patient's social environment. I recommend 5–10 mg of aripiprazole to reduce anxiety and agitation.

Monotherapy should be ideal. But in the case of resistant bipolar disorder, it is not practically possible. On the other hand, the use of more than three agents is harmful due to the risks of synergy and increased side effects, such as cardiac arrest, neuroleptic malignant syndrome, and serotonergic syndrome, which can be life-threatening.

Evidence-based psychotherapy within the setting of cognitive behavioral psychotherapy should be straightforward and available to people with TRSBD. The whole process starts with a psychometric evaluation and an introduction to the possibilities of psychotherapy. The next step is the case formulation, an evidence-based hypothesis that explains, in a simple way, how the issues emerge, how they are kept up, and how they can be dealt with.

ECT is a possible intervention and must be offered by experienced psychiatrists in a setting of a hospital with a psychiatric department. The ECT decision should follow the guidelines of the psychiatric associations. ECT should be offered in treatment-resistant bipolar depression or bipolar mania with psychotic features in cases of severe side effects of the psychiatric agents and of coexistence of other health problems, such as cardiological problems.

A good therapeutic relationship, in which all the issues of agents and their side effects are examined, gives psychiatrists a chance to take after within the long-term execution of pharmacotherapy. Monthly sessions or twice a month display an arrangement for TRSBD in order to upgrade the motivation for taking the agents accurately. Psycho-education, close cooperation with family, and long-term evidence-based psychotherapy and rehabilitation show the proper fixings for successful ambulant therapy for patients with TRSBD.

As the director of the adult psychiatric department of the general hospital "G. Gennimatas" in Athens, Greece, I have followed the above strategy, which has been viable in all my TRSBD cases. It was essential to implement ECT as it were in few cases. So we need to be extremely patient with the advance of our patients with TRSBD and assess them within the long term. Even if ECT is executed, the long-term combination of evidence-based pharmacotherapy and psychotherapy must be carry on.

An ECT that has no success or no impact can devastate the therapeutic relationship and can be characterized as a kind of mishandle. The adherence to agents afterward was exceptionally awful; I had to hospitalize them for 3 months, and the family had misplaced every trust in psychiatry.

So there are always new dimensions in the therapy of TRSBD. A psychiatrist ought to deplete each condition through a combination of evidence-based pharmacotherapy, psychotherapy, and rehabilitation within the setting of a secure, long-term therapeutic relationship.

The clinical psychiatrist must be patient, endorse stable agents suitable for TRSBD, and center not on the fast short-term impact, but on the steady and positive long-term outcome. Hence, compliance with agents will be better. Patients with TRSBD are motivated by the stability and calmness of the psychiatrist and feel secure. We are not permitted to alter the agents in a short period of time, only if it is fundamental. Changes as a result of this treatment will be seen over time. Pharmacotherapy is not a championship in which one must develop triumphant. Pharmacotherapy may be a shared collaboration in which there must be honesty, understanding of any issues, and an open channel of communication for all things. Both sides win when one tunes in to the other. The above is even more critical since pharmacotherapy is the main treatment for TRSBD. It lays the foundation for the usage of the rest of the successful psychotherapies.

The *vulnerability stress model of Zubin and Spring* [37] describes the relationship between vulnerability and stress. High vulnerability under stressful circumstances can lead to relapse (manic, hypomanic, or depressive episode). When vulnerability is decreased, the individual is more competent to cope with stress.

The *cognitive model* considers the vulnerability stress model. A psychological factor that contributes to bipolar disorder, along with biological vulnerability, is the activation of the cognitive triad (the negative beliefs about oneself, others, and the future) [38]. Evaluation of emotional states and dysfunction of emotion regulation strategies contribute to the development of bipolar disorder. The integrative cognitive model shows how appraisals and behaviors interact and contribute to depression and mania.

Positive mood appraisals trigger people with bipolar disorder and lead to mania. It is useful to focus on the cognitive restructuring of positive appraisals of activated mood during a manic phase [39].

The above psychological models present a case formulation for therapy.

Evidence-based psychotherapies for bipolar disorder and treatment-resistant bipolar disorder (bipolar I, bipolar II, cyclothymic disorder) (Fig. 3.1) are accessible. Cognitive Behavioral Psychotherapy (CBT) [1, 38–45], Recovery-Oriented Cognitive Therapy (CT-R) [46], Metacognitive Training (MCT) (www.uke.de/e-mct, www.uke.de/mct_app) [47], various Rehabilitation Programs [48, 49], Recovery-Oriented Therapy Programs, such as the Illness Management and Recovery Program (IMR) [50, 51], psycho-education [1, 52], Cognitive Behavioral Family Therapy [53, 54], Cognitive Behavioral Couple Therapy and Integrative Behavioral Couple Therapy [55–58], and Dialectical Behavior Therapy [59] display the main and most effective psychotherapies for TRSBD (Fig. 3.1).

Psycho-education ought to be combined with the above-mentioned interventions and contribute to increased awareness and insight toward bipolar disorder, which are related to better and longer-term adherence to the treatment, and to effective relapse prevention. A new restart in life is conceivable when people understand their potential and vulnerability in a reasonable setting. In this way, it makes sense for the person to participate in an evidence-based psychotherapy.

CBT contributes to a better coping with depressive, manic, and hypomanic symptoms, which reduces distress from them, and it also contributes to the improvement of anxiety and quality of life. The cognitive restructuring of various schemata, such as the vulnerability, weakness, and grandiosity schemas, presents a key component in this treatment.

CT-R presents the newest development of the Beck Group in the USA for serious mental health disorders. CT-R focuses on activating positive beliefs and actions in the context of TRSBD, which leads to resilience and recovery. Further studies regarding the efficacy of CT-R in bipolar disorder and TRSBD are appropriate.

MCT, a metacognitive intervention, presents a short-term intervention. It is a combination of CBT and rehabilitation, and it can be implemented in a group setting. Individuals with TRSBD pick up more knowledge about cognitive distortions, which are related to depression and mania, and learn to think more realistically. This prevents a potential relapse.

Rehabilitation programs for individuals with TRSBD improve cognitive dysfunction, such as attention, memory, executive function, and functional outcome, which is the key to a better and more realistic reintegration in life.

40–60% of individuals with bipolar disorder show cognitive dysfunction [29]. Participation in a rehabilitation program, which improves cognitive function, makes sense. A good cognitive function provides the basis for the improvement of social function and quality of life.

IMR combines psychoeducation and CBT to enhance the adherence to therapy; it offers also social skills training, the coping of resistant symptoms, and relapse prevention.

Cognitive-behavioral Family Therapy, which evaluates the family dynamic, reduces critical comments or emotional over-involvement of members toward people with TRSBD, improves the communication between them, and rebuilds the dysfunctional schema of the family members.

Cognitive-behavioral Couple Therapy improves, via behavioral interventions, the communication between the partners and engages a new philosophy of the daily coexistence with the taking care program, which focuses on activities that improve the mood of both partners taking care of each other. Afterward, cognitive restructuring of the schemata of both partners with respect to their relationship presents an important cognitive intervention. In other words, active cognitive and behavior change are at the forefront.

Integrative Behavioral Couple Therapy focuses on three strategies in therapy: the affective change enhancing empathy, the cognitive change enhancing a new point of view of the problem, and the behavioral change enhancing new coping with the problem. In other words, emotional acceptance as well as active behavioral change are at the forefront.

Patients with bipolar disorder and TRSBD, who are married or have a stable relationship, need couple therapy, so that the partner can better understand the mood swings and communication problems that arise from depression, mania, and hypomania. A good relationship can improve mood, foster empathy, and prevent suicidality. If the partner of the bipolar patient doesn't know anything about the disorder, this increases the possibility for a divorce during a relapse or during intensive mood swings.

Dialectical behavior therapy improves the main symptoms of bipolar disorder. Further research studies are appropriate [59]. Dialectical behavior therapy regulates the mood swings, helps people accept their own problems without dismissing them, and offers the ability to alter dysfunctional behaviors.

The question is: what ought to be improved for TRSBD? It takes more time to construct a positive therapeutic relationship with these individuals. They feel uncertain, and they are diagnosed with resistant depressive symptoms, manic symptoms, and cognitive dysfunctions. They ought to take all the time they require in order to feel safe before they carry on with the psychotherapy. A majority of them have been treated in an abusive way through polypharmacy or ineffective psychotherapy. In other words, they have lost their belief in mental health experts and are disappointed with everything. This phase increases the possibility of social isolation due to the high burden of stigma and the possibility of dying by suicide.

Motivational interviewing [60] contributes to a better preparation before beginning a psychotherapeutic intervention. The family of the individual ought to be included in this phase and ought to play a positive role in enhancing the motivation of the person with TRSBD.

TRSBD requires long-lasting, recovery-oriented psychotherapy. It is prescribed to combine interventions with each other [61], which ensures the recovery process.

An education in relapse prevention is exceptionally vital in pharmacotherapy and psychotherapy. Individuals with TRSBD learn to evaluate their own mental health status and to cope with changes, which can contribute to relapse. It is very important to take the medication as it is prescribed by the psychiatrist. If a dose is forgotten or if a larger amount of medication is taken, what are the problems? If some side effects arise suddenly, what should be done? It is very important to contact the psychiatrist. If anxiety or a depressive mood arises, then measures should be taken to decrease them, such as doing things that improve the mood or doing sports. If hallucinations or delusions are at the forefront all day and increase anxiety and depression, then interventions should be implemented in order to cope with the hallucination or restructure the delusional thought and all the negative thoughts that are associated with it (Fig. 3.2).

Recovery as an outcome, or objective recovery, means that individuals with TRSBD should be assessed with psychometric tests before, after, and in a follow-up of 6 or more months after the end of the therapy. The results of the tests should reflect the changes-positive, negative, or no changes-after the therapy and in the follow-up.

Recovery as a process, or subjective recovery, means that therapy as a procedure is dynamic, going on, and not at all static. People are responsible for their claimed mental health status and ought to be the protagonists in this context. It can be conceivable that individuals with TRSBD are better psycho-educated after the therapy with respect to their issues; they have diminished their anxiety and manic symptoms, but they require more time to manage successfully with depression.

Some days are easy, and some days are exceptionally troublesome to manage with them. It is necessary to restructure the depressive schema with the negative cognitive triad and the cognitive schema during the manic phase with a positive appraisal of the euphoric and noble state, leading to risky behaviors. In spite of the

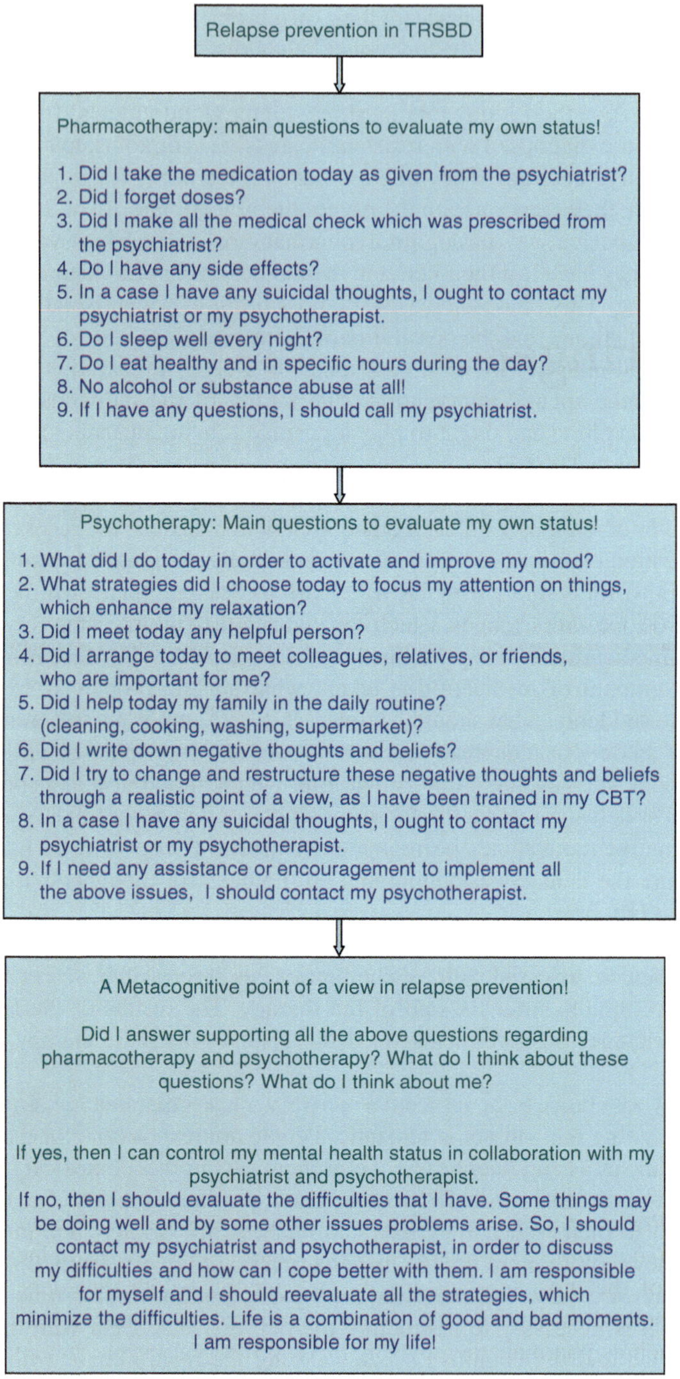

```
┌─────────────────────────────┐
│   Relapse prevention in TRSBD │
└─────────────────────────────┘
                │
                ▼
```

Pharmacotherapy: main questions to evaluate my own status!

1. Did I take the medication today as given from the psychiatrist?
2. Did I forget doses?
3. Did I make all the medical check which was prescribed from the psychiatrist?
4. Do I have any side effects?
5. In a case I have any suicidal thoughts, I ought to contact my psychiatrist or my psychotherapist.
6. Do I sleep well every night?
7. Do I eat healthy and in specific hours during the day?
8. No alcohol or substance abuse at all!
9. If I have any questions, I should call my psychiatrist.

Psychotherapy: Main questions to evaluate my own status!

1. What did I do today in order to activate and improve my mood?
2. What strategies did I choose today to focus my attention on things, which enhance my relaxation?
3. Did I meet today any helpful person?
4. Did I arrange today to meet colleagues, relatives, or friends, who are important for me?
5. Did I help today my family in the daily routine? (cleaning, cooking, washing, supermarket)?
6. Did I write down negative thoughts and beliefs?
7. Did I try to change and restructure these negative thoughts and beliefs through a realistic point of a view, as I have been trained in my CBT?
8. In a case I have any suicidal thoughts, I ought to contact my psychiatrist or my psychotherapist.
9. If I need any assistance or encouragement to implement all the above issues, I should contact my psychotherapist.

A Metacognitive point of a view in relapse prevention!

Did I answer supporting all the above questions regarding pharmacotherapy and psychotherapy? What do I think about these questions? What do I think about me?

If yes, then I can control my mental health status in collaboration with my psychiatrist and psychotherapist.
If no, then I should evaluate the difficulties that I have. Some things may be doing well and by some other issues problems arise. So, I should contact my psychiatrist and psychotherapist, in order to discuss my difficulties and how can I cope better with them. I am responsible for myself and I should reevaluate all the strategies, which minimize the difficulties. Life is a combination of good and bad moments. I am responsible for my life!

Fig. 3.2 A metacognitive model of relapse prevention in TRSBD. Responsibility to myself

fact that there are a few issues, individuals can go on with their lives, whether they are working, studying or assembling friends and family.

Taken together, the main therapy for patients with TRSBD is the evidence-based pharmacotherapy and the cognitive behavioral psychotherapy and rehabilitation. Cognitive behavioral family and couple therapy can also be offered. Dialectical behavior therapy presents also an effective psychotherapy. ECT can be a possible intervention under specific conditions and not for all patients with TRSBD. Psycho-education in relapse prevention presents an important part of the treatment. Lastly, TRSBD require recovery-oriented treatment in a long term.

3.6   Case Studies

All case studies comply with the ethical standards of the 1964 Declaration of Helsinki, and its later amendments, and are presented with permission from TRSBD sufferers. Basic information has been changed to protect individual privacy.

Alexandros is nowadays 35 years old. His psychotherapy was conducted long term in phases over a period of 17 years, with Dr. Rakitzi, with numerous breaks between them. The reason for that was the dynamic change in his psychopathology over the years.

Alexandros participated in a cognitive-behavioral psychotherapy at the age of 19 years between 2007 and 2009. He began to study sociology. At that time, he suffered from panic attacks, major depressive disorder, and an avoidant personality disorder with dependent features. Axis I (panic attacks and major depression episodes) was dealt with as a first priority with behavioral and cognitive interventions in 30 weekly sessions.

A training in assertiveness was systematically implemented, which, in combination with the cognitive restructuring of dependence and avoidance, improved the personality disorder in 40 weekly sessions. One of the main issues during the assertiveness training was how to talk straightforwardly about his homosexuality to other people. He finished his studies and began to work for a non-government organization as a sociologist. He also engaged in a homosexual relationship for many years. Follow-up monthly sessions were done in the next 6 months.

Pharmacotherapy was not given. A psychiatric evaluation was made, but the psychiatrist proposed only systematic psychotherapy. The cooperation with the family was excellent. His parents and his brother supported him a lot and had no problem with his homosexuality. The family's support contributed a lot to the improvement of his mental health.

Psychopathology was assessed through SCL-90-R [20] and DSM-IV-TR [62].

Social skills were evaluated through the Greek version of the German questionnaires FAF (fear of failure) and U (uncertainty questionnaire) [63].

Functional outcome was assessed through the Global Assessment of Functioning (GAF) of the DSM-IV-TR [62].

Anxiety and depression were diminished, and functional outcome was improved (Table 3.1).

Table 3.1 Results of recovery-oriented psychotherapy; psychopathology and functional outcome (2007–2009)

Evaluation	Psychopathology SCL-90-R anxiety T-Score	Psychopathology SCL-90-R depression T-score	Functional outcome GAF
January 2007	$T = 80$	$T = 78$	41
March 2009	$T = 40$	$T = 35$	90

Fear of failure, contact fear, difficulty in saying no, and guilt were diminished and assertiveness was improved. In other words, social skills and assertiveness were improved (Table 3.2).

Alexandros reached Dr. Rakitzi once again in 2012 and asked for a follow-up session. He was very satisfied with his work and wanted to go abroad to a European country to do an M.Sc. in sociology, which would begin in September 2012 and last 1 year. He divorced his partner, and he was trying to make a new beginning in his private life. I suggested he take care of himself for the next period.

Alexandros reached Dr. Rakitzi once more in February 2013. He was disorganized and came back to Athens. He had taken drugs abroad, which induced a psychotic episode in which grandiosity delusion was at the forefront. Alexandros was referred to a psychiatrist for pharmacotherapy. After 1 month, he began once again psychotherapeutic supportive sessions lasting 2 months. The psychotic symptoms retreated after 2 months. After that, Alexandros decided to carry on the therapy with the psychiatrist. I supported this decision because he felt exhausted from this relapse.

Alexandros reached Dr. Rakitzi again in September 2019. He had participated in psychodynamic therapy with another psychotherapist, and he had a relapse. The psychiatrist had prescribed antidepressants. From 2013 until 2019, Alexandros was faced with many treatment-resistant major depressive episodes, which were treated with antidepressants and psychodynamic therapy. In September 2019, he was in a manic episode with grandiosity delusions and substance abuse after a combination of pharmacotherapy and psychodynamic therapy. His parents found another psychiatrist, who changed the medication. A mood stabilizer and antipsychotic agent were prescribed. He was diagnosed with treatment-resistant bipolar I disorder.

Dr. Rakitzi offered him supportive psychotherapy during the manic episode. It took about 3 months to stabilize. A mixed episode with hypomanic and depressive symptoms began in January 2020. He was under pharmacotherapy. He wanted to die by suicide. Dr. Rakitzi cooperated intensively with his family and the psychiatrist to avoid the fulfillment of his suicidal plans. Crisis intervention was at the forefront. The intensity of the suicidal thoughts and plans lasted for 2 months. In March 2020, Dr. Rakitzi started with psychoeducation regarding bipolar disorder and then CBT (30 sessions). The COVID-19 pandemic worsened the situation. In November 2020, Dr. Rakitzi began MCT for bipolar disorder (8 sessions), and I carried on with CT-R from January 2021 until December 2021 (50 sessions). Alexandros had participated in 85 sessions of recovery-oriented psychotherapy, in which CBT, MCT, and CR-T were combined. He accepted his bipolar disorder, he

Table 3.2 Results of recovery-oriented psychotherapy; assertiveness (2007–2009)

Evaluation	Assertiveness FAF	Assertiveness Fear of failure U1	Assertiveness Contact fear U2	Assertiveness Assertiveness U3	Assertiveness Not say no U4	Assertiveness Guilt U5
January 2007	75	57	60	25	40	20
March 2009	30	30	35	45	20	12

Note: *FAF* fear of failure, *U* (uncertainty questionnaire): *U1* fear of failure, *U2* contact fear, *U3* assertiveness, *U4* not say no, *U5* guilt

Table 3.3 Results of recovery-oriented psychotherapy; psychopathology and functional outcome (2020–2021)

Evaluation	SCL-90-R depression T-Score	ARSM scale mania	WHODAS DSM 5 functional outcome
March 2020	80	10	80
December 2021	35	4	30

stopped substance abuse, he found a job for 4 h a day, and he learned to appreciate his life, finding new goals.

Depression was assessed through the SCL-90-R [20] and DSM-5 [64], mania through the Altman self-rating mania scale [65] and DSM 5 [64], and finally, functional outcome through WHODAS [22, 23].

Depression and mania were diminished, and he was more stabilized. The functional outcome was improved (Table 3.3). The combination of evidence-based pharmacotherapy and psychotherapy was effective for Alexandros.

The above case shows how a psychopathology can be created over time. A therapeutic relationship was constructed up from the primary treatment between 2007 and 2009. This contributed to the fact that Alexandros came back for a new intervention in the context of cognitive-behavioral therapy. He portrayed the psychodynamic therapy as something that was appealing at the beginning, but it has driven him to chaos at the cognitive and behavioral levels. The cooperation with his family and his psychiatrist was excellent. These days, Alexandros is under pharmacotherapy, has accepted his bipolar I disorder, and works for a family company.

Athina began a cognitive-behavioral psychotherapy with Dr. S. Rakitzi in January 2005 after the reference of her psychiatrist. She showed self-destructive behaviors-engravings in her arms and legs with a razor blade, suicide attempts with pills, which led to hospitalizations, resistant suicidal thoughts and plans, excessive alcohol consumption, binge-eating episodes, and a hypersexual behavior. She was sexually abused when she was 15 years old! Furthermore she was diagnosed with borderline personality disorder. She was hospitalized five times and had monthly ambulant psychiatric treatment. The psychiatrist prescribed venlafaxine 150 mg, risperidone 1 mg and alprazolam 0.5 mg and changed the doses in relation to the problems. Athina didn't see any progress with the pharmacotherapy. Dr. Rakitzi gave the following diagnosis: Axis I Panic disorder, bipolar disorder I, and Axis II borderline personality disorder. During the therapy, it was clear that a dual diagnosis of borderline personality disorder and bipolar I disorder was the biggest problem! This was clearer in 2006.

Cognitive-behavioral psychotherapy in combination with dialectical behavior therapy and pharmacotherapy was offered between January 2005 and October 2006 once a week. She completed 96 CBT sessions.

She learned to manage her panic attacks and her depression, and after that, we focus on self-destructive behaviors, borderline personality disorder, and mood swings. CBT and dialectical behavior therapy contributed a lot to the decrease of suicidality, to decrease of spending large amounts of money, of alcohol consume, of binge-eating episodes, and of hypersexual behavior. She married her partner and wanted to be a mother.

The following psychometric evaluations were made: psychopathology was assessed through SCL-90-R [20] and DSM-IV-TR [62]. Social skills were evaluated through the Greek version of the German questionnaire U (uncertainty question-naire) [63]. January 2005: Anxiety $T = 80$ (SCL-90-R), Depression $T = 85$ (SCL-90-R), GAF 41, U (fear of failure 60, assertiveness 22, not say no 42). October 2006: Anxiety $T = 50$, Depression 57, GAF 90, U (fair of failure 32, assertiveness 45, not say no 22). Athina held monthly follow-up sessions between October 2006 and December 2006. The improvement was very clear. She married and worked many hours. Psychiatric treatment was carried on.

All these years, I have cooperated with her parents and her husband in order to help them understand Athina, her self-destructive behavior, and her mood swings! Athina is very lucky to have such as a supportive family.

In spring 2009, Athina had called; she was in crisis and wanted to die by suicide. She took her medication, but she didn't perceive any improvement! She took venla-faxine 150 mg, alprazolam 1 mg, and interrupted risperidone. Likewise, she has taken drugs (cocaine), drunk a lot of alcohol, and had hypersexual behavior. She was in a manic episode. I propose a hospitalization.

I refer her and her family to Dr. Georgila, who was at the time director of the psychiatric department of the general hospital "G. Gennimatas" in Athens, Greece, and who also proposed hospitalization. Dr. Georgila stopped venlafaxine 150 mg and gave 900 mg lithium and 15 mg olanzapine. She was stabilized after 6 months ambulant psychiatric treatment. Dr. Georgila continued with the treatment of Athina until today and gave the following agents: lithium 900 mg, citalopram 20 mg, and clozapine 150 mg. Nowadays, clozapine 150 mg and citalopram 40 mg are being given. Clozapine helps Athina mostly! Nowadays, Athina is the mother of two chil-dren and is under control with the guidance of Dr. Georgila, receiving psychiatric treatment every 2 months. Depression was assessed through the SCL-90-R [20] and DSM 5 [64], mania through the Altman self-rating mania scale [65] and DSM 5 [64], and finally, functional outcome through WHODAS 2 weeks ago [22, 23]. Depression $T = 50$ (SCL-90-R), mania 4 (ARSM scale) and functional outcome 20 (WHODAS). Recovery has been in process for Athina all these years!

Athina wrote a letter to borderline personality disorder and bipolar disorder,

Dear borderline personality disorder and bipolar disorder,

I have spent many hours during my life with my mood swings, with my suicidal-ity, with psychiatrists and clinical psychologists. I leave a life out of limits and with no control. I took many bad risks during my life, and it is a miracle that I didn't die. My neurotransmitter and my psychological traumas contributed to my psychopathology.

The negative moments began with impulsive behavior, self-destructive behav-ior, and panic attacks in a depressive or maniac phase. I have two selves. When I am in a manic phase, I think that I can achieve everything and that I am a woman with special abilities. Life is wonderful. When I am in a depressive phase, I want to die. I cannot value my life. I have tried all the agents in psychiatry. Some psychiatrists prescribed me seven agents for every day. After many years of psychiatric treatment and psychotherapy, I have learned to cope with panic, with my depression, and to avoid self-destructive behaviors and we have found the medication that helped very much, leponex (clozapine). My resistant interest in dying has stopped with clozapine.

I married, and we decided after 8 years to have children. I now have twins, a boy and a girl. My children help me every day to have specific goals and to do as many things as possible so that they can be happy! My life has changed positively after many years of self-destructive behaviors. I know now that I can cope with my treatment-resistant bipolar disorder.

George is 45 years and has been a one-handed disabled person since birth and suffers from treatment-resistant bipolar disorder. His mother also suffered from it. Dr. Georgila has treated him for 10 years and has been hospitalized many times. The following agents have been given: Lithium and olanzapine, lithium, olanzapine and citalopram, valproate 1200 mg, clozapine 250 mg, and amisulpride 200 mg. George had suffered from many manic episodes with rapid mood fluctuations, great anxiety, and resistant agitation.

Elena is 74 years old and has suffered from treatment-resistant bipolar disorder since she was 20 years old. She worked in academia. Dr. Georgila treated her 10 years. Antidepressants, lithium, and atypical antipsychotics were prescribed for 3 years without efficacy in functional outcome. Parkinson was diagnosed by a neurologist in the last 5 years, and many relapses have arisen in the last 3 years. Therefore, pharmacotherapy was changed to lithium and clozapine in combination with antiparkinsonism agents (Madopar). In the last 2 years, lithium was stopped due to kidney failure, and clozapine remained (150 mg) with quetiapine (100 mg). In 1 year, a bowel cancer diagnosis was given, which led to more mood fluctuations and, lastly, a resistant depressive state. This woman has no family support, and she is neglected by her family.

Nikos is 52 years old. He is treated 20 years. He suffers from treatment-resistant bipolar II disorder. He takes the following agents: Venlafaxine 150 mg, olanzapine 10 mg, and valproate 1000 mg. Nikos suffers from treatment-resistant depression. Dr. Georgila has changed the medication many times due to resistant depressive phases and hypomanic phases. Treatment-resistant depression is a situation in which we must change many antidepressant agents. There is a danger of manic phases with venlafaxine. The mood stabilizer is very crucial and should be given.

Kalliopi, is 41 years old, works part-time, has no children, and is not married. She is treated by Dr. Georgila. She had three manic episodes followed by mild depressive episodes with poor adherence to medication. Mania was expressed with episodes of weekly insomnia, agitation, slurred speech or gonorrhea with negative exposure to the work and family environment. She usually suffers 1 month from mania and then 4 months from depression. Olanzapine 20 mg was given due to poor compliance, Dr. Georgila gave her long-acting injectable agent aripiprazole 400 mg in combination with olanzapine 7.5 mg. Mania and depression phases have been normalized for a year now. Her functional outcome has improved a lot.

Nikos is today 74 years old. He has been treated by psychiatrists since he was 25 years old. He was diagnosed as patient with schizophrenia. He was treated in the age of 25–30 years old by psychiatrists of a famous psychiatric department in Athens, Greece, between 1980 and 1994 with many and high doses of antipsychotics who recommended afterward also ECT. Nikos participated in 120 sessions of ECT and during that period, he wanted to die by suicide. This terrible situation led him and the family to visit another psychiatric department in Athens, the psychiatric department of the general hospital G. Gennimatas in Athens, Greece. Dr. Georgila treated Nikos in cooperation with Prof. Garellis, who was the director of the psychiatric department of the General hospital "G. Gennimatas" in Athens, Greece. ECT was not necessary and Nikos was also misdiagnosed. He didn't suffer from schizophrenia. He suffered from an atypical affective disorder.

He was treated for many years until today by Dr. Georgila who prescribed, during the year's minitran 2 mg and then antidepressants. Dr. Georgila offered him cognitive behavioral psychotherapy. Today, Nikos is 74 years old. He has suffered from leukoencephalopathy since 1 year and he is treated with escitalopram (10 mg), clonazepam (1 mg), and quetiapine (300 mg).

There were also cases that showed great difficulty in cooperating.

Maria wanted to begin a structured cognitive-behavioral psychotherapy. She was in a depressive phase. She participated in psychoanalytic therapy for 10 years that was terminated. This led to a manic episode. A long-term cognitive behavioral therapy of 50 sessions was proposed and explained how it could be effective for her bipolar disorder. She was very exhausted from the psychoanalytic therapy and has decided to carry on only with pharmacotherapy.

Manos wanted to begin with a cognitive behavioral psychotherapy. He was in a manic phase and had interrupted his pharmacotherapy. He didn't want to have any contact with his psychiatrist. A psycho-education was offered in order to enhance his motivation to begin his pharmacotherapy again. A cognitive-behavioral psychotherapy in a manic phase without pharmacotherapy is not possible to be offered and can be dangerous. Manos has been referred to another psychiatrist.

The following conclusions can be drawn from the above case studies:

A stable therapeutic relationship with the clinical psychiatrist as well as with the clinical psychologist and cognitive behavioral psychotherapist is important for a safe diagnosis and treatment.

Treatment-resistant bipolar disorder is underestimated or under diagnosed or misdiagnosed.

The diagnosis must be entered safely. If a manic episode exists, then it enters more easily. If a first depressive episode arises, it takes longer to make a potential diagnosis of bipolar disorder. Misdiagnosis of bipolar disorder with schizophrenia and psychotic disorders is a very common phenomenon.

This leads to the fact that large doses of antipsychotic agents are being given without being necessary, with a lot of stigmas and a lot of bad side effects, such as the metabolic syndrome.

Hospitalization can be necessary in manic and severe depressive episodes.

Early diagnosis of resistant bipolar disorder prevents bad events, such as suicide.

Long-acting injectable agents can help increase pharmacotherapy compliance.

Cooperation with the family and supportive environment (spouse, partner) is essential. Psycho-education of the family and spouse or partner in the disorder is essential.

The combination of pharmacotherapy and cognitive behavioral psychotherapy in depression in bipolar disorder I, II and cyclothymia and in the hypomanic phase (bipolar II, cyclothymia) is very effective.

ECT should be offered under specific conditions, and specifically in treatment-resistant depression and treatment-resistant manic phase with psychotic features, if the agents are not effective and cause serious health problems, such as cardiological problems.

Pharmacotherapy is the main intervention in the manic phase of bipolar I disorder. Only supportive psychotherapeutic treatment is recommended, not systematic psychotherapy of any kind.

Cognitive behavioral psychotherapy during a hypomanic phase is not recommended. Psychiatric treatment is the main treatment and after the impact of agents in about 2 months, cognitive behavioral psychotherapy can be implemented.

The diagnosis of PTSD in bipolar disorders is also a common phenomenon. Particularly in bipolar I and II disorders, exposure to trauma should be avoided, and cognitive interventions should be followed to deal with the psychological effects of trauma (physical, sexual, and verbal-emotional abuse). Exposure to trauma can lead to a severe depressive or manic episode.

The comorbidity of borderline personality disorder and bipolar disorder is a very common phenomenon and makes both pharmacotherapy and cognitive behavioral psychotherapy difficult.

The comorbidity of bipolar disorder and substance abuse also complicates treatment and requires multilevel interventions from both pharmacotherapy and cognitive behavioral psychotherapy.

A large percentage of bipolar patients with substance abuse disorder and borderline personality disorder have a large possibility of belonging to the TRSBD category.

The percentage of patients with TRSBD who seeks help from a psychiatrist or a cognitive-behavioral psychotherapist is very small and that is why we have a high relapse rate in TRSBD.

If patients with TRSBD have participated in a non-evidence-based psychotherapy, it can be possible that they are not enough motivated to begin with a new psychotherapy or that they don't trust any more psychotherapies.

Taken together, all the above cases have shown that evidence-based pharmacotherapy and cognitive-behavioral psychotherapy are effective for TRSBD. The comorbidity of bipolar disorder and borderline personality disorder present one of the most difficult issues. Systematic cognitive behavioral psychotherapy during a manic phase is not recommended. The sooner the diagnosis of TRSBD is being given, the better for the patients with TRSBD. Finally, TRSBD is under diagnosed or misdiagnosed.

3.7   Discussion

8 million adults in the USA and 40 million individuals worldwide suffer from bipolar disorder. 75% of the symptomatic phase contains depression or depressive symptoms. Diagnosis and therapy are delayed by approximately 9 years. More than 50% show very poor adherence to treatment, and life expectancy is reduced due to other organic problems, such as the metabolic syndrome and type 2 diabetes. 15–20% of people with bipolar disorder die by suicide. Antidepressants, but not as monotherapy, mood stabilizers, and antipsychotic agents are recommended in pharmacotherapy. Psycho-education, cognitive-behavioral psychotherapy, cognitive behavioral family therapy, and cognitive-behavioral couple therapy are the psychotherapies of first choice for individuals with bipolar disorder [66, 67].

Bipolar disorder is a severe mental health disorder. TRBD presents a chronic mental health disorder that is related to persistent manic, hypomanic, and depressive symptoms, persistent cognitive dysfunctions, more hospitalizations, resistant suicidal behavior, poor adherence to pharmacotherapy and psychotherapy, and a diminished quality of life.

Resistant cognitive dysfunctions burden the daily routine and increase the depressive and manic symptoms, and vice versa. Patients with TRSBD are desperate under these conditions, which can increase suicidality. They are trapped in a vicious circle of weakness, a dead end and without perspective. This decreases the adherence to pharmacotherapy and increases the possibility of hospitalization, a relapse, and social isolation.

TRSBD is frequently underestimated or under diagnosed or misdiagnosed. It takes healing time to understand the existence of the disorder. On the other hand, knowledge and experience can help in the correct diagnostic assessment.

The comorbidity of bipolar disorder with substance abuse and borderline personality disorder should activate experts to make a better differential diagnosis. This condition increases the possibility of the existence of TRSBD which can lead to a higher percentage of suicidality.

Nowadays, it cannot be blamed that TRSBD is something obscure! The sooner it is recognized, the better for the patients and their families.

The therapeutic relationship with patients with TRSBD and their families presents a very interesting level of involvement. It enacts the resources of mental health experts within the long term. It could be an exceptionally intensive setting that empowers us to be motivated for changes and new adaptations in life. When patients with TRSBD and their families are seeking out a new mental health expert, we listen the same history: they have been hospitalized numerous times after extreme relapses, they have poor adherence to pharmacotherapy, they have misplaced their believe in science and they want to die by suicide.

It is additionally exceptionally common to have a secondary benefit from TRSBD: patients have all the consideration of the family on them; they don't ought to attempt a lot because family solves problems in cases where interfamily relations are great. In this manner, we require evidence-based interventions to teach them to go from an addictive and symbiotic relationship with the family to more independence from segregation and depression as a result of stigma to more activity for life and from cognitive dysfunction to way better concentration, memory and problem-solving.

So we require to grant them sufficient time and space to precise themselves and make with them a new commitment: we show them a new way of coping with their mental health disorder and be the protagonist of their own life. Their family is additionally desperate and has no hope for something superior in the future. The family ought to be the portion of the treatment and contribute to the numerous and critical changes. If the family behaves competitively and doesn't coordinate with the mental health experts, we ought to center on our cooperation with the patients with TRSBD.

Transparency, professionalism, and evidence-based interventions are the proper fixings for building a safe and secure therapeutic relationship. A transparent explanation regarding evidence-based pharmacotherapy, psychotherapy, and rehabilitation builds trust and persuades patients and their families to embrace new dimensions of life.

The therapeutic relationship shows a motivational context that empowers mental health experts to be confident toward sufferers of TRSBD, so that they can alter step- by step issues that have an incredible negative impact on functional outcomes. This assertive context activates a dynamic interpersonal therapeutic relationship that gives life a new meaning in life.

We go from suicidal crisis, loneliness, despair, weakness, confinement, and stigma to hope, self-responsibility toward their possess issues, cohesive connections with mental health experts and the family, and finally, activation of their own resources to manage every hour, every day, every week, every month, and every year with TRSBD. This procedure gives life a new meaning.

The therapeutic goals should be straightforward within the setting of the therapeutic relationship. Side effects of pharmacotherapy and polypharmacy ought to be treated as a first priority. This circumstance diminishes the plausibility of suicidal risk and bad adherence to pharmacotherapy. The following step ought to be the treatment of depressive and manic symptoms as well as cognitive dysfunctions, which incorporates a positive impact on functional outcomes.

Nowadays, we can construct up a suitable therapeutic plan with respect to the combination of evidence-based interventions and treat all the therapeutic objectives.

The majority of patients with TRSBD display treatment-resistant cognitive dysfunctions. Cognitive dysfunctions are categorized in neurocognitive dysfunctions (information processing speed, concentration, working memory, memory, problem-solving) and in social cognitive dysfunctions (theory of mind, attribution, social perception, social knowledge). Neurocognitive and social cognitive dysfunctions are distinct categories.

ECT can be an alternative after the failure of the appropriate pharmacotherapy with serious side effects, such as cardiological problems, in treatment-resistant depression and mania with psychotic features Nevertheless, this decision ought to be considered. Cost and benefits of ECT should always be taken into consideration.

The comorbidity of TRSBD and severe personality disorder should be treated with special care. TRSBD with avoidant, dependent, obsessive- compulsive, schizotypal and narcissistic personality disorders can participate in an individual setting as well as in a group setting with other personality disorders without many obstacles. TRSBD with obsessive-compulsive disorder and obsessive-compulsive personality disorder displays a difficult case that takes longer to stabilize and to build an appropriate therapeutic relationship. On the other hand, it is possible to participate in a group therapy without many difficulties.

TRSBD with borderline, histrionic, schizoid and antisocial personality disorders have more problems in a group setting. It is recommended to begin with those personality disorders with an individual cognitive-behavioral therapy and try to carry on with group cognitive-behavioral therapy and rehabilitation. If this is not possible, it is recommended to carry on with an individual cognitive behavioral therapy for bipolar disorder and personality disorders.

Antisocial personality disorder doesn't respect others and their rights, and it shows criminal behavior many times. Schizoid prefers lonely activities; histrionic seek always intensive attention; and borderline personality disorder shows unstable and impulsive behavior all the time. All these parameters decrease the possibility of remaining in a group psychotherapeutic setting.

Severe personality disorders should be treated according to the cognitive-behavioral model of Beck [68]. Interventions on the level of personality that focuses on the restructure of the main schemas of the personality disorder contribute to an increase in functional outcomes in the daily routine.

On the other side, if TRSBD is being treated properly, this could also have a positive impact also on the personality disorder. TRSBD is the main diagnosis on which we should focus the therapy. Personality disorder should be treated after the stabilization of TRSBD.

The combination of TRSBD and borderline personality disorder antisocial, schizoid, and histrionic personality disorder is one of the most difficult, according to clinical experience. An antisocial personality disorder doesn't accept the rules of society. These people destroy every interpersonal relationship and are dangerous, showing criminal behavior. A borderline personality disorder shows impulsive, unstable, and auto- destructive behavior. If this impulsive behavior is affected by the psychotic symptoms, such as hallucinations, this is a very critical situation. A schizoid prefers lonely activities, and this increases the possibility coming to a group therapy. A histrionic personality seeks for attention all the time! So, it is very important to have them in an individual setting of cognitive behavioral therapy and rehabilitation for TRSBD and personality disorders, and afterward to propose that they participate in a group setting with other members having the same problems, such as TRSBD and borderline, antisocial, schizoid, and histrionic personality disorder.

The presented case studies showed the complexity and difficulties as well as the chances of TRSBD treatment. Suicidality is the first priority for these patients. Negative experiences regarding side effects with agents, polypharmacy or not-necessary ECT, and non-evidence-based psychotherapy and rehabilitation should be discussed openly without steoreotypes and avoidant strategies from mental health experts.

RECOVERYTRSBDGR, a recovery-oriented program that is talked about in Chap. 4, offers a really seriously treatment with numerous sessions. Patients with TRSBD, who come to take part in it, regularly have other experiences with other colleagues.

A central message ought to be sent: A democratic society is responsible for protecting vulnerable people by appearing ways of being assertive toward their rights or the infringement of their rights. This setting will help sufferers from TRSBD and their families to construct a new and steady therapeutic relationship with the mental health experts that will lead to a new restart of the treatment. A long-term combination of evidence-based interventions regarding pharmacotherapy, psychotherapy, and rehabilitation is the only way to a new restart in life. The experience of physical, psychological, and sexual abuse by patients with TRSBD makes the therapy more difficult and our responsibility toward them bigger. Especially, the abuse from mental health experts is the most troublesome circumstance for all of us. It is additionally one of the most unethical behavior in our profession. Exposure to trauma is not recommended.

All the evidence-based interventions for TRSBD (psychoeducation, CBT, CR-T, rehabilitation) ought to be implemented so that the schemas of loss of control, weakness, vulnerability, and abandonment as a consequence of the trauma can be restructured.

Case studies showed that evidence-based interventions for TRSBD are nowadays available. As mental health experts, we ought to update our education regarding these interventions and to make these modern treatments known to the community through books, journal papers, participation in conferences, workshops, and other social media.

Private and public mental health departments should be evaluated to determine whether evidence-based interventions are being offered and how effective and efficacious their execution is.

Living with TRSBD and a chronic mental health disorder means the enactment of a grief process, which ought to be communicated. Denial, anger, bargaining, depression, and acceptance are the five stages of the grief process that are communicated by means of depressive or manic symptoms regarding the coexistence of a chronic mental health disorder. Clinical psychiatrists and clinical psychologists ought to be very careful with those phases that are associated with high suicidal risk and bad adherence to pharmacotherapy.

The patients with TRSBD and their families endure from an intensive grief process throughtout their lives. It takes time to acknowledge a long-term vulnerability with negative consequences for your entire life.

Individual psychiatric treatment and individual sessions of cognitive-behavioral psychotherapy are essential dealing with the grief process. Family sessions are also recommended if all the family members suffer at the same time from active grief. It is very troublesome to fight with such a disorder with so many consequences on emotional, behavioral, and cognitive levels and on quality of life. Patients with TRSBD and their families ought to have the opportunity to express their grief in a safe and structured psychotherapeutic setting. This confrontation with the grief leads to depression in the short term but prepares the road to a long term and new restart in life. The sooner the grief process is being treated, the better for the sufferers from TRSBD.

Patients with TRSBD understand that this disorder has a strong biological basis and, in combination with psychological vulnerability, can lead to a relapse. In other words, patients with TRSBD understand that pharmacotherapy is the main therapy, and without it, a relapse is very conceivable. The participation on a combination of evidence-based psychotherapy and rehabilitation is the next step.

The long-term participation in evidence-based treatments transforms the grief process into an action for life, for improvement and for a new reintegration into society and a new restart in life. The grief process can be activated in any phase of the lives of people with TRSBD and their families. Long-term action against TRSBD through evidence-based interventions is the best way to express this grief.

Recovery-oriented interventions lead patients with TRSBD and their families from the long-term grief process to action for step-by step improvement in the daily routine and to action for gaining more objectives in life.

Stigma as a consequence of a chronic mental health disorder is something that can be a central issue in the treatment. Patients with TRSBD feel embarrassed, disconnected, and this decreases the possibility for seeking for professional help. The society stigmatizes patients with TRSBD and their families. So, a secure and steady therapeutic relationship in the context of a long-term recovery-oriented therapy will contribute to a restructuring of schemas that are associated with the stigma.

The long-term intervention, in which treatments will be combined, will lead to steady ambulant treatment with stable reference persons-therapists. Fixed ambulant places build a home and a family! Whatever bad happens, these frameworks are there to absorb crises and pave the way for recovery.

The long-term therapeutic relationship will go through difficult and pleasant moments. The main denominator of all is communication around issues that make everyday life difficult and increase dysfunctional behavior. The compass of the therapeutic relationship is the evidence-based interventions and how these are applied at the appropriate level.

Mental health professionals must be dedicated to their work in arrange to do their best to accompany patients with TRSBD and their families with dignity, professionalism and efficiency. Finally, this long-term therapeutic relationship is a very beautiful journey. It is an honor for experts to have this role in the lives of our vulnerable fellow citizens.

Mental health experts must never forget what TRSBD means: there are specific pharmacotherapies that are recommended; psychotherapy must be long term, combine various interventions and at the same time, give the possibility of repeating them.

Individuals with TRSBD are often traumatized by the difficulties that arise over the years. They are regularly faced with a postponed diagnosis of TRSBD, with numerous phenomena of non-evidence-based pharmacotherapy and polypharmacy, and non- evidence-based psychotherapy, which doesn't improve symptoms, increases suicidality, and diminishes quality of life. This situation leads to misplaced trust and belief, and more suspiciousness toward treatments. Mental health experts ought to acknowledge the above behaviors at the beginning of therapy and should try to win the trust of these people in the context of evidence-based pharmacotherapy and psychotherapy.

The percentage of patients with TRSBD who seek psychotherapy spontaneously is very small. This can be explained by the fact that they have been fighting with their problems for many years, with many hospitalizations and relapses, which have led to a decrease in trust in treatments.

Clinical psychiatrists and clinical psychologists should inform the society via conferences and books what TRSBD is and how it can be managed. This book will try to fill this gap and give more information about TRSBD and its treatment.

Psycho-education, the appropriate pharmacotherapy for TRSBD without the phenomenon of polypharmacy, and a long-term recovery-oriented psychotherapy are the steps that develop a new therapeutic relationship characterized by more trust, hope, mutual understanding, transparency, and more democracy and respect toward the human rights of individuals with TRSBD.

They should understand the meaning of TRSBD, the difficulties that arise from it, and how important it is to take specific medications and to be under a recovery-oriented psychotherapy.

The diagnosis must be entered safely. Using an agent would be the best solution. Resistant bipolar disorder, unfortunately, does not allow this. On the other hand, the use of more than three agents is harmful and lead to unwanted side effects.

Psycho-education, CBT, CR-T, rehabilitation programs, MCT, cognitive behavioral family therapy, cognitive behavioral couple therapy, and recovery programs present evidence-based psychotherapies for TRSBD. Relapse prevention ought to always be included in evidence-based psychotherapies. Further studies regarding the effectiveness and efficacy of the above interventions in TRSBD are appropriate.

Further research regarding the efficacy of evidence-based pharmacotherapy and psychotherapy in a difficult diagnostic category, such as TRSBD, is required.

When people with TRSBD are faced with psychological traumas, such as abuse, at that point, it is prescribed not to execute exposure to trauma, but to work more with cognitive interventions in the context of CBT and CR-T, which lead to a diminishment of the severity of schemas regarding vulnerability, weakness, and loneliness and increase positive beliefs about self, others, and the future, enhancing resilience.

MCT can improve symptoms, cognitive functions, and quality of life through a metacognitive perspective. Afterward, an integrative rehabilitation program that improves symptoms, cognitive functions, social skills and problem-solving can improve reintegration into society. Recovery programs, cognitive behavioral family therapy, and cognitive behavioral couple therapy can also support reintegration into society and a feeling of security in this world. After all these interventions by people with TRSBD and traumas, life starts to be more secure, with a higher quality of life and a new meaning of life.

Individuals with TRSBD appear to have resistant depressive, manic, and hypomanic symptoms and cognitive dysfunctions, as well as high suicidal risk. That means that long-term, recovery-oriented pharmacotherapy and psychotherapy ought to be given. It is well known that people with TRSBD require more time to improve their quality of life. The use of a combination of many different psychotherapies at numerous levels, such as individual therapy, group therapy, family therapy, and couple therapy, with a possible repetition of them after 1 or 2 years, is the most suitable way to treat resistance in bipolar disorder. The repertoire of the available interventions is large enough to combine different and numerous evidence-based psychotherapies.

The therapeutic relationship and alliance plays an important role in combination with interventions in the context of cognitive-behavioral psychotherapy and rehabilitation. This relationship is characterized by empathy, acceptance, support under every condition, and therapeutic limits.

Patients with TRSBD are inspired by the therapeutic relationship to express their thoughts and feelings without shame or guilt and to talk about many potential forms of abuse, such as physical, sexual, and psychological abuse during their life and the traumas of suicidality, polypharmacy, and the implementation of non-evidence-based psychotherapies. A supportive therapeutic relationship is open toward all difficult issues, such as suicidality. If patients want to die by suicide, they know that they can talk about it in the therapy, and this fact decreases the social isolation and the possibility of dying by a suicide! They can lean on this important therapeutic relationship in order to think more realistic and to find possible alternative solutions by their own lives.

Recovery as an outcome and recovery as a process should be two diverse points of views, which must be taken into thought for the assessment of the result of the reintegration into society of the individuals with TRSBD.

What should be done in the future? Effective pharmacotherapy without polypharmacy and side effects is now required for TRSBD. A combination of evidence-based interventions in the context of CBT and rehabilitation with the possibility of a repetition of psychotherapy presents the treatment of choice for TRSBD, which ought to be a fundamental goal in research protocols in the future.

Taken together, TRSBD presents a severe chronic mental health disorder with a high percentage of suicidal risk. The sooner it is recognized, the better for the patients and their families. The long-term therapeutic relationship is a very important element implementing evidence-based pharmacotherapy and psychotherapy. The treatment of depression, mania–hypomania, cognitive dysfunctions, stigma, and grief are the main elements of the evidence-based interventions. The comorbidity of TRSBD with severe personality disorders and TRSBD with psychological traumas should be taken carefully into consideration in the treatment.

3.8 Conclusions

Bipolar disorder and TRSBD are severe chronic mental health disorders. TRSBD is associated with high suicidal risk. Evidence-based and recovery-oriented pharmacotherapy and psychotherapy are the treatments of first choice. Relapse prevention should also be an integral part of the treatment. Case studies displayed the significance of the recovery-oriented treatments.

Revision Questions

1. Please characterize bipolar disorder.
2. Please define TRSBD.
3. Why is TRSBD troublesome?
4. Evidence-based pharmacotherapy for TRSBD.
5. Evidence-based psychotherapy for TRSBD.
6. What should be done to improve evidence-based pharmacotherapy and psychotherapy in TRSBD?
7. Please depict and clarify the recovery as an outcome and the recovery as a process in TRSBD.
8. Please depict the metacognitive model of relapse prevention in TRSBD.
9. Which components with respect to TRSBD ought to be in the center of research in the future?

Competing Interests   The authors have no conflicts of interest to declare that are relevant to the content of this chapter.

Ethical Approval   Our case studies follow the ethical standards of the 1964 Declaration of Helsinki. Informed consent to publish was obtained from individual participants.

The authors offer approximately once a year a course about the evidence-based treatments of CBT and rehabilitation for treatment-resistant bipolar disorder for clinical psychologists, clinical psychiatrists, and cognitive behavioral psychotherapists. For more information, please see https://www.linkedin.com/in/stavroula-rakitzi-0b512b45/, http://orcid.org/0000-0002-5231-6619 (Stavroula Rakitzi), https://gr.linkedin.com/in/polyxeni-georgila-940b521a7, http://orcid.org/0000-0003-3137-506x (Polyxeni Georgila) or email srakitzi@gmail.com.

References

1. Yatham LN, Kennedy SH, Parikh SV, Schaffer A, Bond DJ, Frey BN, Sharma V, Goldstein BI, et al. Canadian Network for Mood and Anxiety Treatments (CANMAT) and International Society for Bipolar Disorders (ISBD) 2018 guidelines for the management of patients with bipolar disorder. Bipolar Disord. 2018;20:97–170. https://doi.org/10.1111/bdi.12609.
2. Fountoulakis KN, Grunze H, Vieta E, Young A, Yatham L, Blier P, Kasper S, Moeller HJ. The international college of neuro-psychopharmacology (CINPN) treatment guidelines for bipolar disorder in adults (CINP-BD-2017), part 3: the clinical guidelines. Intern J Neuropsychopharm. 2017;20(2):180–95. https://doi.org/10.1093/ijnp/pyw109.
3. Howes OD, Thase ME, Pillinger T. Treatment resistance in psychiatry: state of the art and new directions. Mol Psychiatry. 2022;27:58–72. https://doi.org/10.1038/s41380-021-01200-3.
4. Diaz AP, Fernandes BS, Quevedo J, Sanches M, Soares JC. Treatment-resistant bipolar depression: concepts and challenges for novel interventions. Braz J Psychiatry. 2022;44(2):178–86. https://doi.org/10.1590/1516-44462020-1627.
5. Kessler U, Schoeven HK, Vaaler AE, Andreassen OA, Eide GE, Hammar A, Malt UF, Oedegaard KJ, et al. Neurocognitive profiles in treatment-resistant bipolar I and bipolar II disorder depression. BMC Psychiatry. 2013;13:105. https://doi.org/10.1186/1471-244x-13-105.
6. Sanches M, Bauer IE, Galvez JF, Zunta-Soares GB, Soares JC. The management of cognitive impairment in bipolar disorder: current status and perspectives. Am J Ther. 2015;22(6):477–86. https://doi.org/10.1097/MJT.0000000000000120.

7. Scheepstra KWF, van Doorn JB, Scheepens DS, de Haan A, Schukking N, Zantvoord B, Lok A. Rapid speed of response to ECT in bipolar depression: a chart review. J Psychiatry Res. 2022;147:34–8. https://doi.org/10.1016/j.jpsychires.2022.01.008.

8. Salagre E, Rohde C, Vieta E, Østergaard SD. Electroconvulsive therapy following incident bipolar disorder: when, how, and for whom? Bipolar Disord. 2022;24:817–25. https://doi.org/10.1111/bdi.13254.

9. Mutz J. Brain stimulation treatment for bipolar disorder. Bipolar Disord. 2023;25:9–24. https://doi.org/10.1111/bdi.13283.

10. Perugi G, Medda P, Toni C, Mariani MG, Socci C, Mauri M. The role of electroconvulsive therapy (ECT) in bipolar disorder: effectiveness in 522 patients with bipolar depression, mixed state, mania and catatonic features. Curr Neuropharmacol. 2017;15:359–71. https://doi.org/10.2174/1570159X14666161017233642.

11. American Psychiatric Association. Diagnostic and statistical manual of mental disorders. DSM 5-TR. Washington: American Psychiatric Publishing; 2022.

12. Perugi G, Hantouche E, Vannucchi G. Diagnosis and treatment of cyclothymia: the primacy of temperament. Curr Neuropharmacol. 2017;15:372–9. https://doi.org/10.2174/1570159X14666160616120157.

13. Rosenblat JD, McIntyre RS. Treatment of mixed features in bipolar disorder. CNS Spectr. 2017;22(2):141–6. https://doi.org/10.1017/s1092852916000547.

14. Shobassy A. Elderly bipolar disorder. Curr Psychiatry Rep. 2021;23(5):5. https://doi.org/10.1007/s11920-020-01216-6.

15. Correa R, Akiskal H, Gilmer W, Nierrenberg AA, Trivedi M, Zisoak S. Is unrecognized bipolar disorder a frequent contributor to apparent treatment resistant depression? J Affect Disord. 2010;127(1-3):10–8. https://doi.org/10.1016/j.jad.2010.06.036.

16. Aas M, Henry C, Andreassen OA, Bellivier F, Melle I, Etain B. The role of childhood trauma in bipolar disorders. Int J Bipol Disor. 2016;4:2. https://doi.org/10.1186/s40345-015-0042-0.

17. Miller CJ, Johnson SL, Eisner L. Assessment tools for adult bipolar disorder. Clin Psychol. 2009;16(2):188–201. https://doi.org/10.1111/j.1468-2850.2009.01158.x.

18. Bech P. Rating scales for psychopathology, health status and quality of life. Berlin: Springer; 1993. p. 325–40.

19. Fountoulakis KN, Iacovides A, Kleanthous S, Samolis S, Gougoulias K, Kaprinis G, Bech P. The Greek translation of the symptoms rating scale for depression and anxiety: preliminary results of the validation study. BMC Psychiatry. 2003;3:21. http://www.biomedcentral.com/1471-244X/3/21.

20. Donias S, Karastergiou A, Manos N. Standardization of the symptom checklist-90-R rating scale in a Greek population. Psychiatrist. 1991;2(1):42–8.

21. Haddock G, McCarron J, Tarrier N, Faragher EB. Scales to measure dimensions of hallucinations and delusions: the psychotic symptom rating scales (PSYRATS). Psychol Med. 1999;29(4):879–89.

22. World Health Organization. International classification of functioning, disability and health (ICF). Geneva: World Health Organization; 2001.

23. Koumpouros Y, Papageorgiou E, Sakellari E, et al. Adaptation and psychometric properties evaluation of the Greek version of WHODAS 2.0. pilot application in Greek elderly population. Heal Ser Out Res Methods. 2018;18(1):63–74. https://doi.org/10.1007/s10742-017-0176-x.

24. Hancock N, Scanlan JN, Bundy AC, Honey A. Recovery assessment scale–domains & stages (RAS-DS) manual-version 3. Sydney: University of Sydney; 2019.

25. Hancock N, Rakitzi S, Katoudi S. Recovery assessment scale-domains & stages (RAS-DS). The Greek version; 2023.

26. Hancock N, Scanlan J, Honey A, Bundy A, O'Shea K. Recovery assessment scale – domains & stages (RAS-DS): its feasibility and outcome measurement capacity. Austr N Z J Psychiatry. 2015;49(7):624633. https://doi.org/10.1177/0004867414564084.

27. Parker GB, Graham RK. Clinical characteristics associated with treatment resistant bipolar disorder. J Nerv Ment Dis. 2017;205(3):188–91. https://doi.org/10.1097/NMD.0000000000000517.

28. Spoorthy MS, Chakrabarti S, Grover S. Comorbidity of anxiety and bipolar disorders: an overview of trends in research. World J Psychiatry. 2019;9(1):7–29. https://doi.org/10.5498/wjp.v9.i1.7.
29. Sole B, Jimenez E, Torrent C, Reinares M, del Mar Bonnin C, Torres I, et al. Cognitive impairment in bipolar disorder: treatment and prevention strategies. Int J Neuropsychopharmacol. 2017;20(8):670–80. https://doi.org/10.1093/ijnp/pyx032.
30. Di Florio A, Craddock N, van den Bree M. Alcohol misuse in bipolar disorder. A systematic review and meta-analysis of comorbidity rates. Eur Psychiatry. 2014;29(3):117–24. https://doi.org/10.1016/jeuropsy.2013.07.004.
31. Preuss UW, Schefer M, Born C, Grunze H. Bipolar disorder and comorbid use of illicit substances. Medicina. 2021;57(11):1256. https://doi.org/10.3390/medicina57111256.
32. Zimmerman M, Morgan TA. The relationship between borderline personality disorder and bipolar disorder. Dialogues Clin Neurosci. 2013;15(2):155–69. https://doi.org/10.31887/DCNS.2013.15.2/Zimmermann.
33. Poon SH, Sim K, Baldessarini RJ. Pharmacological approaches for treatment-resistant bipolar disorder. Curr Neuropharmacol. 2015;13:592–604.
34. Wilkowska A, Cubala WJ. Clozapine as transformative treatment in bipolar patients. Neuropsychiat Dis Treatment. 2019;15:2901–5. https://doi.org/10.2147/NDT.S227196.
35. Delgado A, Velosa J, Zhang J, Dursun SM, Kapczinski F, de Azevedo CT. Clozapine in bipolar disorder: a systematic review and meta-analysis. J Psychiatry Res. 2020;125:21–7. https://doi.org/10.1016/j.jpsychires.2020.02.026. Epub 2020 Feb. 27.PMID: 32182485.
36. Katz IR, Rogers MR, Lew R, Thwin SS, Doros G, Aheam E, Ostacher MJ, DeLisi LE, Smith EG, et al. Lithium treatment in the prevention of repeat suicide-related outcomes in veterans with major depression or bipolar. Disord JAMA Psychiatry. 2022;79(1):1–10. https://doi.org/10.1001/jamapsychiatry.2021.3170.
37. Zubin J, Spring BJ. Vulnerability – a new view of schizophrenia. J Abnorm Psychol. 1977;86:103–26.
38. Beck AT. Cognitive therapy and the emotional disorders. New York: International University Press; 1976.
39. Palmier-Claus JE, Dodd A, Tai S, Emsley R, Mansell W. Appraisals to affect: testing the integrative cognitive model of bipolar disorder. Br J Clin Psychol. 2016;55(3):225–35. https://doi.org/10.1111/bjc.12081.
40. Newman CF, Leahy RL, Beck AT, Reilly-Harrington NA, Gyulai L. Bipolar disorder. A cognitive therapy approach. Washington: American Psychological Association; 2003.
41. Chiang KJ, Tsai JC, Liu D, Lin CH, Chiu HL, Chou KR. Efficacy of cognitive-behavioral therapy in patients with bipolar disorder: a meta-analysis of randomized controlled trials. PLoS One. 2017;12(5):e0176849. https://doi.org/10.1371/journal.pone.0176849.
42. Baldessarini RJ. Evidence-based options for treatment resistant adult bipolar disorder patients. Bipolar Disord. 2012;13:573–84. https://doi.org/10.1111/j.1399-5618-2012.01042.x.
43. Hofmann SG, Asnaani A, Vonk IJJ, Sawyer AT, Fang A. The efficacy of cognitive behavioral therapy: a review of meta-analyses. Cogn Ther Res. 2012;36(5):427–40. https://doi.org/10.1007/s10608-012-9476-1.
44. Scott J, Bentall R, Kinderman P, Morriss R. Is cognitive behaviour therapy applicapble to individuals diagnosed with bipolar depression or suboptimal mood stabilizer treatment: a secondary analysis of a large pragmatic effectiveness trila. Int J Bipol Disord. 2022;10:13. https://doi.org/10.1186/s40345-022-00259-3.
45. Novick DM, Swartz HA. Evidence-based psychotherapies for bipolar disorder. Focus. 2019;17:238–48. https://doi.org/10.1176/appi.focus.20190004.
46. Beck AT, Grant P, Inverso E, Brinen AP, Perivoliotis D. Recovery oriented cognitive therapy for serious mental health conditions. New York: The Guilford Press; 2021.
47. Haffner P, Quinlivan E, Fiebig J, Sondergeld LM, Strasser ES, Adli M, et al. Improving functional outcome in bipolar disorder: a pilot study on meta cognitive training. Clin Psychol Psychother. 2018;25(1):50–8.
48. Palumbo D, Mucci A, Giordano GM, Piegari G, Aiello C, Pietrafesa D, Annarumma N, Chieffi M, Cella M, Galderisi S. The efficacy, feasibility and acceptability of a remotely accessible

use of CIRCuiTs. A computerized cognitive remediation therapy program for schizophrenia: a pilot study. Neuropsych Diseas Treat. 2019;15:3103–13. https://doi.org/10.2147/NDT.S221690.

49. Torrent C, del Mar Bonnin C, Marinez-Aran A, Valle J, Amann BL, Gonzalez-Pinto A, Crespo JM, Ibanez A, et al. Efficacy of functional remediation in bipolar disorder: a multicenter randomized controlled study. Am J Psychiatry. 2013;170:852–9.

50. Mueser KT, Meyer PS, Penn DL, Clancy R, Clancy DM, Salyers MP. The illness management and recovery program: rationale, development and preliminary findings. Schizophr Bull. 2006;1:32–43. https://doi.org/10.1093/schbul/sbl022.

51. McGuire AB, Kukla M, Green A, Gilbride D, Mueser KT, Salyers MP. Illness management and recovery. A review of the literature. Psychiatry Serv. 2014;65(2):171–9. https://doi.org/10.1176/appi.ps.201200274.

52. Rabelo JL, Cruz BF, Ferreira JDR, de Mattos Viana B, Barbosa IG. Psycho education in bipolar disorder. World J Psychiatry. 2021;11(12):1407–24. https://doi.org/10.5498/wjp.v11.i12.1407.

53. Hutcheson CL. Cognitive behavioral family therapy. In: Metcalf L, editor. Marriage and family therapy. A practice-oriented approach. Cham: Springer; 2019. p. 95–118.

54. Samar BS, Akkus K, Kutuk B. Effectiveness of cognitive behavioral family therapy: a systematic review of randomized controlled trials. Curr Approaches Psychiatry. 2023;15(1):175–88. https://doi.org/10.18863/pgy.1115301.

55. Fischer MS, Baucom DH, Cohen MJ. Cognitive behavioral couple therapies: review of the evidence for the treatment of relationship distress, psychopathology and chronic health conditions. Fam Process. 2016;55(3):423–42. https://doi.org/10.1111/famp.12227.

56. Christensen A, Doss BD. Integrative behavioral couple therapy. Curr Opin Psychol. 2017;13:111–4. https://doi.org/10.1016/j.copsyc.2016.04.022.

57. Christensen A, Doss BD, Jacobson NS. Integrative behavioral couple therapy. A therapist guide to creating acceptance and change. New York: Norton & Company; 2020.

58. Baucom BR, Atkins DC, Simpson LE, Christensen A. Prediction of treatment response at 5-year follow-up in a randomized clinical trial of behaviorally based couple therapies. J Consult Clin Psychol. 2015;83:103–14.

59. Jones BDM, Umer M, Husain MI. A systematic review on the effectiveness of dialectical behavior therapy for improving mood symptoms in bipolar disorders. Int J Bipol Disord. 2023;11:6. https://doi.org/10.1186/s40345-023-00288-6.

60. Miller WR, Rollnick S. Motivational interviewing: preparing people for change. New York: The Guilford Press; 2002.

61. Rakitzi S. Clinical psychology and cognitive behavioral psychotherapy. recovery in mental health. Cham: Springer; 2023.

62. American Psychiatric Association. DSM-IV-TR diagnostic criteria. Athens: Medical Publications of Litsa; 2004.

63. Αντωνίου Β, Ευθυμίου Κ, Μυλωνά Κ. Κοινωνικό άγχος, διεκδικητικότητα και κοινωνική φοβία. In: Ένα δομημένο ομαδικό πρόγραμμα γνωσιακής συμπεριφοριστικής θεραπείας. Αθήνα: ΙΕΘΣ; 2015.

64. American Psychiatric Association. Diagnostic and statistical manual of mental disorders. DSM 5. Washington: American Psychiatric Publishing; 2013.

65. Altman EG, Hedeker D, Peterson JL, Davis M. The Altman self-rating mania scale. Soc Biol Psychiatry. 1997;42:948–55.

66. Nierenberg AA, Agustini B, Köhler-Forsberg O, Cusin C, Katz D, Sylvia LG, Peters A, Berk M. Diagnosis and treatment of bipolar disorder. A review. JAMA. 2023;330(14):1370–80. https://doi.org/10.1001/jama.2023.18588.

67. Hirschfeld RMA, Bowden CL, Gitlin M, Keck PE, Suppes T, Thase ME, Wagner ME, Perlis RH. Practice guideline for the treatment of patients with bipolar disorder. 2nd ed. Washington: American Psychiatric Association; 2010.

68. Beck AT, Freeman A, Davis DD. Cognitive therapy of personality disorders. New York: The Guilford Press; 2004.

A New Recovery-Oriented Treatment Model for Treatment-Resistant Bipolar Disorder

4

Learning Objectives
1. A new recovery-oriented pharmacotherapy for TRSBD.
2. A new recovery-oriented psychotherapy for TRSBD.
3. Advantages and disadvantages of this new model.

4.1   Introduction

The long clinical experience and collaboration of Dr. S. Rakitzi and Dr. P. Georgila led them to develop a recovery-focused therapy model for TRSBD (bipolar I, bipolar II, cyclothymic disorder). TRSBD is associated with high suicide rates, more cognitive dysfunction, more hospitalizations, and frequent relapses. All of these variables have contributed to the development of a new recovery-oriented model.

The Greek health system has many structural problems. The mental health system in Greece is multidimensional; various psychotherapies are applied, but without evaluating their effectiveness. Patients with TRSBD go from hospital to hospital without having done systematic therapeutic work that will deal with the problem at its root. Thus, there was a need to create a structured and effective model for TRSBD.

Additionally, the disappointment of patients with TRSBD, their long-term grief, their frustration, and the continued suicidal crisis have motivated us to focus on the development of a structured and evidence-based program for TRSBD in which patients and their families are included in a collaborative context.

Long-term participation in such a program can lead sufferers of TRSBD to work systematically with problems and to find a new meaning in life with more resilience and hope.

There are well-known etiological models of bipolar disorder that were considered in our model.

S. Rakitzi, P. Georgila, *Treatment-Resistant Bipolar Disorder*, https://doi.org/10.1007/978-3-031-59001-6_4

The following neurotransmitters contribute to the pathogenesis of bipolar disorder: *noradrenaline, serotonin, dopamine, and gamma-aminobutyric acid*. Abnormal activity of the hypothalamic-pituitary-adrenal cortex has been registered in bipolar disorder [1].

Zubin and Spring's [2] *vulnerability-stress model* describes the relationship between vulnerability and stress. High vulnerability in stressful situations can lead to relapse. Vulnerability factors may include discontinuation of pharmacotherapy, emotional over- involvement or behavior of rejection by family members toward the person with TRSBD, alcohol and substance abuse, or lack of sleep. Stress is something that's continuously displayed, for example, due to financial problems, unemployment or the death of a loved one. When vulnerability is controlled or reduced, individuals become more capable of adapting to stress.

The cognitive model considers the vulnerability-stress model. A psychological factor that contributes to bipolar disorder, along with biological vulnerability, is the activation of the cognitive triad (the negative beliefs about self, others, and the future) [3].

Evaluation of emotional states and dysfunction of emotion regulation strategies contribute to the development of bipolar disorder. The integrative cognitive model shows how appraisals and behaviors interact and contribute to depression and mania. Positive mood appraisals trigger people with bipolar disorder and lead to mania [4].

Psychometric tests, such as the symptom checklist 90-R [5], the Altman self-rating Mania Scale [6] for symptoms, the Symptoms Rating Scale for Depression and Anxiety (SRSDSA) [7, 8], and the psychotic symptom rating scales (PSYRATS) [9], can also be used.

WHODAS 2. 0 [10, 11] for disability and functional capacity and the Recovery Assessment Scale-Domains and Stages (RAS-DS) for the evaluation of the recovery process [12, 13] offer valid and reliable tests, and they should be performed before, after treatment, and at follow-up 6 months. WAIS [14] should be used before treatment to show the burden of cognitive dysfunction and intellectual ability, and it is repeatable after 1 year.

An intelligence quotient (IQ) $\geq$ 80 is a necessary condition to participate in our recovery model for TRSBD. Selection criteria: *inclusion criteria:* age 18–65, IQ $\geq$ 80, diagnosis TRSBD. *Exclusion criteria:* Substance abuse and head injuries. If substance abuse is successfully treated, the participant will be acknowledged into our program.

Our clinical experience with TRSBD has shown us the path to effective therapy for these people: *long-term recovery-oriented* pharmacotherapy and psychotherapy, with the possibility of *repeating* the treatment procedure. Individuals with TRSBD require more time to reset after negative experiences and construct trust in the scientific community.

Well-known and evidence-based psychological therapies in individual and group settings, such as CBT [15], CR-T [16], and MCT [17] are included and recommended because of their effectiveness and efficacy for people with bipolar disorders and their worldwide acknowledgment within the international community. We are exceptionally thankful to the creators of the above therapies, such as Dr. A. Beck and his colleagues and Prof. S. Moritz and his colleagues, who have made these treatments accessible to the scientific community.

Finally, our proposal for implementing these psychotherapies in RECOVERYTRSBDGR (Fig. 4.1) presents the results of our clinical experience with them over the years and our recognition of their value and adequacy in clinical practice.

A. Introductory phase (3 months) (20 sessions)
   Psychometric evaluation regarding intelligence, symptoms, functional outcome and recovery before the intervention (recovery as an outcome).

1. Month: (8 sessions) two individual sessions of one hour per week, one session with the clinical psychiatrist and one session with the clinical psychologist and cognitive behavioral psychotherapist. Build of therapeutic relationship, psycho-education, motivational interviewing, negative past experiences with treatments.

2. Month: (4 sessions) one individual session of 90 minutes per week together with the clinical psychiatrist and clinical psychologist and cognitive behavioral psychotherapist. Build of therapeutic relationship, psycho-education to the family and reduction of high-expressed emotion, motivational interviewing.

3. Month: (8 sessions) two individual sessions of one hour per week with the clinical psychiatrist and clinical psychologist and cognitive behavioral psychotherapist. Build of therapeutic relationship, psycho-education, motivational interviewing and enhancement of assertiveness to claim their rights.

B. Second phase (108 sessions)

1. Individual psychotherapy (cognitive phase) (100 sessions)
   CBT (30 sessions) (once a week 1 hour), CR-T (70 sessions) (once a week, one hour)

2. A pause of 2 months

3. Group psychotherapy (metacognitive phase) (8 sessions)
   MCT (8 sessions) (once a week, each one hour).

C. Third phase (2 months) (8 sessions) (Epilogue)

1 individual follow-up session weekly of 90 minutes together with the clinical psychiatrist and clinical psychologist and cognitive behavioral psychotherapist and with the person with TRSBD and the family. Relapse prevention. Recovery as a process.

D. 4 monthly individual sessions are being given as follow-up.

Total number of sessions of RECOVERYTRSBDGR: 140.

E. Psychometric evaluation regarding symptoms, functional outcome and recovery after the intervention (recovery as an outcome).

F. Psychometric evaluation regarding symptoms, functional outcome and recovery in a follow-up after six months (recovery as an outcome).

E. Recommendation for cognitive-behavioral couple therapy after the completion of RECOVERYTRSBDGR.

Fig. 4.1 Recovery-oriented pharmacotherapy and psychotherapy for people with TRSBD. A Greek model (RECOVERYTRSBDGR)

There are three points of view that play a central role in our model (RECOVERYTRSBDGR) (Fig. 4.1). The cognitive perspective that centers on our cognition (thoughts, beliefs, and schema), the metacognitive perspective, which is awareness of thoughts, beliefs, and schemata (thoughts about cognitions), and the recovery perspective that centers on recovery as an outcome or objective recovery and recovery as a process or subjective recovery.

Our recovery-oriented therapy (RECOVERYTRSBDGR) (Fig. 4.1) consists of three phases: introduction, recovery-oriented therapy, and conclusion. The second phase includes a combination of evidence-based pharmacotherapy, cognitive behavioral psychotherapy, and metacognitive intervention. Known and evidence-based psychotherapies are incorporated first in the context of *individual therapy (the cognitive phase)* and second in the context of *group therapy (the metacognitive phase)*.

RECOVERYTRSBDGR (Fig. 4.1) contributes to the balance of neurotransmitters responsible for bipolar disorder by improving insight, symptoms, cognitive function, restructuring cognitive distortions related to delusions and hallucinations, improving family communication, as well as functional outcomes and recovery.

RECOVERYTRSBDGR (Fig. 4.1) aims to be executed in the coming years in Greece and other countries and help as many individuals with TRSBD as conceivable.

In sum, the problems in the Greek health system as well as the problems with patients with TRSBD have motivated us to develop a structured and evidence-based recovery-oriented program. Our model is based on specific etiological models that are considered in our model. Inclusion and exclusion criteria for patients with TRSBD and the psychometric tests that can be used are described. RECOVERYTRSBDGR consists of three phases: introduction, recovery-oriented therapy, and epilogue. Evidence-based pharmacotherapy and psychotherapy are being offered. Finally, three perspectives—the cognitive, the metacognitive, and the recovery perspective play an important role.

4.2   Recovery-Oriented Pharmacotherapy for Bipolar Disorder and Treatment-Resistant Bipolar Disorder (P. Georgila)

The first phase of this model is the introductory phase, which is carried out by all mental health professionals responsible for the recovery process of the person with TRSBD (clinical psychiatrist, clinical psychologist, cognitive-behavioral psychotherapist). This first phase includes 3 months of treatment. Psychological assessment will be performed before intervention with respect to intellectual quotient, symptoms, functional outcome, and recovery process.

During the *first month, four individual sessions* are committed to build the therapeutic relationship, conducting motivational interviews, and providing psychoeducation around TRSBD and the significance of pharmacotherapy. Two 1-h sessions per week are offered, one with a clinical psychiatrist and one with a clinical psychologist and cognitive-behavioral psychotherapist.

During the *second month, four weekly sessions* of 90 min each with a clinical psychiatrist, clinical psychologist, and cognitive-behavioral psychotherapist are devoted to building therapeutic relationship, motivational interviewing, and psychoeducation by the family of the person with TRSBD, so that the importance of pharmacotherapy and psychotherapy can be examined and the high expressed emotion of the members can be decreased.

Finally, in the *third month, two individual 1-h sessions per week*—one with a clinical psychiatrist and a second with a clinical psychologist and cognitive-behavioral psychotherapist—are additionally given to the therapeutic relationship, motivational interviewing on the importance of pharmacotherapy and psychotherapy, and discourse of potential issues with the family of the person with TRSBD. An introduction to recovery-oriented psychotherapy will be displayed. Psychiatrists and psychologists must inform individuals with TRSBD of all their rights and how they can claim them. For example, individuals with TRSBD have the right to receive financial support from the government and support through employment. Non-evidence-based pharmacological treatment (polypharmacy) and non-evidence-based psychotherapy ought to be avoided. If they are victims of misconduct, mental health professionals should help them look for legal help.

Mood stabilizers, antipsychotics, and antidepressants are the main combinations of agents in TRSBD. Pharmacotherapy should be adjusted, which depends on whether we have bipolar I, bipolar II disorder or a cyclothymia and on which phase the patients are—depressive, manic, or hypomanic phase. Pharmacotherapy should be chosen in favor of patients with TRSBD with fewer side effects and satisfied remission and recovery.

Patients are ready after a minimum of 3 months of readjustment of the agents to start with the RECOVERYTRSBD. It will not be possible to participate in RECOVERYTRSBD in a resistant manic phase, which needs intensive psychiatric treatment and cooperation with the family.

The third phase (epilogue) of RECOVERYTRSBDGR keeps going for *2 months*. Clinical psychiatrists, clinical psychologists, and psychotherapists work together to supply weekly individual 90-min follow-up sessions for people with TRSBD and their families to see the effect of the second stage of RECOVERYTRSBDGR and to relieve the strong emotions of family members. Repeating the process will yield a better assessment.

Finally, *four individual monthly sessions* are offered for follow-up.

In sum, the pharmacotherapy in the context of RECOVERYTRSBDGR has been described. Pharmacotherapy is the main therapy, which is the main condition, so that evidence-based psychotherapy can be implemented. A new restart in pharmacotherapy after many unsuccessful sessions of pharmacotherapy in the past is not an easy choice. The clinical experience of psychiatrists is in demand.

4.3   Recovery-Oriented Cognitive-Behavioral Psychotherapy and Metacognitive Training for Bipolar Disorder and Treatment-Resistant Bipolar Disorder (S. Rakitzi)

The first phase of this model is the introductory phase and is carried out by all mental health professionals responsible for the recovery process of the person with TRSBD (clinical psychiatrist, clinical psychologist, cognitive-behavioral psychotherapist).

This *first phase* includes *3 months* of treatment. Psychological assessment will be performed before intervention regarding intellectual quotient, symptoms, cognitive function, functional outcome, and recovery process.

During the *first month, eight weekly individual 1-h sessions* are devoted to building the therapeutic relationship, conducting motivational interviewing, carrying out psychoeducation around TRSBD and the significance of psychotherapy. Two sessions per week are offered, one with a clinical psychiatrist and one with a clinical psychologist and cognitive-behavioral psychotherapist.

During the *second month, four weekly sessions of 90 min* each with a clinical psychiatrist, clinical psychologist, and cognitive-behavioral psychotherapist are devoted to building therapeutic relationships, motivational interviewing, and carrying out psychoeducation by the family of the person with TRSBD, to be able to discuss the significance of psychotherapy and reduce the emotions that members express presently.

Finally, in the *third month, eight sessions—two individual 1-h sessions per week*—one with a clinical psychiatrist and the second with a clinical psychologist and cognitive psychotherapist—are additionally committed to the therapeutic relationship, motivational interviewing on the importance of pharmacotherapy and psychotherapy, and examining potential issues within the family of the individual with TRSBD.

A presentation on recovery-oriented psychotherapy will be displayed. Psychiatrists and psychologists must advise people with TRSBD of all their rights and how they can claim them. For example, people with TRSBD have the right to receive financial support from the government and support through employment. Non-evidence-based pharmacological treatment (polypharmacy) and non-evidence-based psychotherapy ought to be avoided. If they are victims of unfortunate behavior, mental health professionals should help them seek legal help.

Motivational interviewing may be a specific style of communication and collaboration within the therapeutic relationship that centers on change. The pros and cons of potential changes are discussed. People with specific mental health disorders and TRSBD have expanded motivation to change in the context of acceptance and commitment. Motivational interviewing incorporates four processes:

(1) Engaging: developing a working relationship, (2) Focusing: Develop a focus on change during the conversation, (3) Evoking: discussing the motivation for change, (4) Planning: develop a commitment to change and a specific plan of action [18]. Non-adherence to medication treatment and low motivation in psychotherapy

can be discussed in motivational interviewing, so that people with TRSBD can discover new points of view on pharmacotherapy and psychotherapy.

Taken together, the primary 3 months represent an *introductory phase* aimed at building the therapeutic relationship and restarting with adequate, evidence-based pharmacotherapy. If suicidal thoughts or plans are progressing, a cognitive-behavioral intervention particularly related to suicidal ideation should be executed, as described in the following paragraphs.

The first part of the *second phase* of RECOVERYTRSBDGR centers on a long-term combination of evidence-based pharmacotherapy and psychotherapy for people with TRSBD. The *first phase* of psychotherapy focuses on *individual therapy (the cognitive phase)* and a combination of evidence-based individual psychotherapies. The following psychotherapies are prescribed: individual CBT therapy at a rate of 30 weekly 1-h sessions and CR-T 70 weekly 1-h sessions to better adapt with symptoms and the resulting distress and reinforce positive beliefs about yourself, which can have a positive impact on managing symptoms. Suicide should be the primary issue that must be talked about and settled in CBT. We talk about it straightforwardly and teach people how to bargain with it. After 100 sessions, there is a 2-month break to unwind and see the impacts of psychotherapy. Psychiatric treatment takes place once a month.

It is exceptionally important to begin with individual psychotherapy so that people have time to progress and to specifize their challenges. It is well known that people with TRSBD are exceptionally suspicious and traumatized by frequent and ineffective treatments in the past! This means they first need individual psychotherapy to gain confidence in evidence-based treatments and prepare for the second part, which focuses on group psychotherapy.

Suicidal behavior must be treated with a preventative and restorative approach, with openness and transparency, and without stereotypes. It is very important to talk about this issue with all people with TRSBD, notwithstanding whether they are currently actively suicidal or not. Most of them have confronted it in the past; indeed, on the off chance that they don't have it right now.

A good therapeutic relationship will provide a secure setting to talk transparently about the issue and react with empathy and renewed hope. A transparent psycho-educational approach to suicidal behavior by portraying thoughts and behaviors and displaying an intervention structure against it and for more hope in life contributes to more straightforwardness, security and control of troublesome circumstances. Suicidal therapy is conveyed within the context of a cohesive and collaborative therapeutic relationship.

The Five-Step Suicide Assessment and Triage (SAFE-T) (www.sprc.org or www.stopasuicide.org) displays a very effective framework for mental health professionals, which incorporates numerous factors that can be evaluated in full detail and significance. The following steps are prescribed: (1) Identify risk factors. (2) Identify protective factors. (3) Suicide investigation (suicidal thoughts, plans, behaviors and intent). (4) Evaluation of risk and choice of the appropriate intervention to cope with the risk, and finally, (5) Documentation (evaluation of risk, intervention and follow-up).

A suicide prevention contract must be signed between a clinical psychiatrist, clinical psychologist, and cognitive-behavioral psychotherapist and the individual with TRSBD and suicidal thoughts. The individual can contact mental health experts to cope with the suicidal thoughts, intentions, and plans and to arrange sessions with a clinical psychiatrist and clinical psychologist as soon as possible. The above contract diminishes impulses toward suicide and social isolation while also sending a central message: people with TRSBD are not alone and can continuously discover other ways to cope with hallucinations, delusions, depression, and despair.

People with TRSBD and suicidal thoughts and behavior feel vulnerable, weak within to confront of bipolar disorder, isolated and stigmatized, and with luck of control on the disorder. Individuals with TRSBD are often depleted by bipolar disorder, have a destitute quality of life, and have no other options in this life but suicide.

CBT is a compelling treatment for suicidal tendencies and contributes to diminishing suicidal ideation attempts [19].

CBT educates people with TRSBD about cognitive interventions and especially about not accepting automatic thoughts related to suicidal ideation as reality. These automatic thoughts are linked to basic cognitive schemas, such as vulnerability, weakness, loneliness, and abandonment. People with TRSBD feel very isolated. CBT trains them to cope with the manic and depressive symptoms and thus control them. Then, gradually, they feel less vulnerable, weak, and lonely, and they have more control over TRSBD and their own lives. CR-T can enhance positive self-beliefs about the ability to cope with bipolar disorder and the ability to see new perspectives and meaning in life.

The family of a person with TRSBD must be informed about the potential danger of suicidal thoughts and attempts if the person has a good relationship with the family and if the family is aware of the person's TRSBD. Psychoeducation about TRSBD and suicidal ideation plays an important role.

The latter part of the *second phase* of the combination of evidence-based pharmacotherapy and psychotherapy centers on the combination of *group* evidence-based programs *(rehabilitation and metacognitive phase),* which focus on cognitive distortions that are related to bipolar disorder. MCT for bipolar disorder for eight sessions once a week for 1 h. Eight sessions will be offered during this second phase of psychotherapy.

MCT will be provided by a clinical psychiatrist, a clinical psychologist and cognitive- behavioral psychotherapist, trained in this program. Psychiatric treatment takes place once a month.

The third phase (epilogue) (eight sessions) of RECOVERYTRSBDGR lasts 2 months. Clinical psychiatrists, clinical psychologists, and psychotherapists work together to provide weekly, 1-h individual follow-up sessions for people with TRSBD and their families to see the impact of the second stage of RECOVERYTRSBDGR and reduce the strong emotions of family members. Psychoeducation on relapse prevention will be provided. Repeating the process will yield a better assessment. The recovery perspective (recovery as a process or subjective recovery) plays an important role in this third phase (epilogue) and is a central theme of the sessions.

Recovery as an outcome or objective recovery means that individuals with TRSBD should be evaluated with psychometric tests before, after, and in a follow-up period of 6 or more months after the end of the therapy.

Recovery as a process or subjective recovery means therapy as a dynamic and ongoing procedure rather than static. Individuals must take responsibility for their own mental health and be protagonists. For example, it may be that people with TRSBD have improved in many areas, such as anxiety and depression, but they need more time to cope effectively with manic phases.

Finally, *four individual monthly sessions* are offered for follow-up. These sessions are held in collaboration with clinical psychiatrists, clinical psychologists, and people with TRSBD.

Psychological assessments regarding symptoms, functional outcomes, and recovery will be performed after completion of RECOVERYTRSBDGR and at 6-month follow-up. Psychiatric treatment takes place once a month. If relapse occurs after 12 months, the combination of pharmacotherapy and evidence-based psychotherapy (RECOVERYTRSBDGR) above should be repeated.

A cognitive-behavioral couple therapy can be implemented after RECOVERYTRSBDGR on the off chance that TRSBD is responsible for potential problems within the marriage.

Taken together, the implementation of evidence-based psychotherapy in the context of RECOVERYTRSBDGR has been described and explained. Suicidal risk should be treated as a priority before RECOVERYTRSBDGR is offered. 140 sessions will be offered in total. It is possible to repeat the whole program if the results are not satisfactory or a relapse has taken place.

4.4   Discussion

TRSBD is associated with high burden and poor quality of life. Our experience with TRSBD led us to think about developing a new recovery-oriented model in which all constraints are taken into consideration. TRSBD requires long-term recovery-oriented and evidence-based pharmacotherapy and psychotherapy.

Nowadays, preparing the conditions to incorporate evidence-based treatments is extremely important [20].

Suicidal risk is one of the greatest issues for patients with TRSBD. In this way, it is the primary need for any therapeutic intervention. Altering medication, working with the family, and engaging in evidence-based interventions are the most excellent choices. Suicidal risk could be a result of discontinuation of medication, improper regulation of bipolar disorder, or TRSBD. Patients feel sad, they don't see any electives or ways out of their life and they don't discover any meaning in their lives.

Antidepressants, mood stabilizers, and antipsychotic agents are the main categories of agents used to treat TRSBD. Bipolar I, II and cyclothymia present different categories and the pharmacotherapy should be adjusted appropriately. The sooner TRSBD is being treated properly with agents, the smaller the possibility for suicidality.

Pharmacotherapy needs a minimum of 3 months to reach a good level and to see potential side effects. A good therapeutic relationship and alliance with the psychiatrist is appropriate in order to discuss openly and with honest every problem.

When patients are stabilized with the appropriate combination of agents, we can carry on with the combination of pharmacotherapy and RECOVERYTRSBDGR.

The introduction phase of RECOVERYTRSBDGR tries to enroll negative experiences and contributes to a new restart in the context of evidence-based treatments. The second phase provides effective evidence-based individual and group psychotherapies. The conclusion may be a survey of all the changes that have been made and changes related to the quality of life of patients with TRSBD and their families. Finally, 4 monthly follow-ups aim to separate and assess recovery or subjective recovery. Psychiatric treatment is the main therapy and takes place once a month. Individual and group psychotherapy within the framework of cognitive-behavioral psychotherapy and metacognitive intervention is an adjunct therapy to pharmacotherapy. A psychological assessment will be given pre-intervention, post-intervention, and at 6-month follow-up (recovery as an outcome). A cognitive-behavioral couple therapy can be implemented after RECOVERYTRSBDGR when potential problems within the marriage arise.

RECOVERYTRSBDGR (Fig. 4.1) endures 140 sessions and instructs people with TRSBD and their families how to cope with bipolar disorder and suicidal risk, improve symptoms, recovery, and achieve functional outcome results. People find new meaning in life after a troublesome diagnosis. People learn to allude to a stable therapy group for help. This ambulatory setting minimizes the probability of hospitalization and increases the likelihood of living in the community in the context of social reintegration focused on recovery. This program is advertised to individuals with treatment-resistant bipolar I, bipolar II, and cyclothymic disorder.

Mental health professionals ought to devote themselves to this therapy over the long term and over many years. This implies they must have clinical experience and appropriate training for the long-term treatment of chronic mental health disorders, such as bipolar disorder.

RECOVERYTRSBDGR (Fig. 4.1) has advantages and disadvantages. Its benefit is that it is a recovery-oriented therapy that includes evidence-based treatments for people with TRSBD; it secures people from repeated hospitalizations and suicidal behavior; it offers the possibility of rehashing the program after 12 months in case of relapse; and it may be a good example of the significance of good cooperation between a clinical psychiatrist and clinical psychologist. Cognitive and metacognitive perspectives are taken into consideration. Recovery as an outcome and recovery as a process are critical parts of this therapy.

Taken together, RECOVERYTRSBDGR presents an overview of evidence-based treatments in TRSBD. The disadvantages are that the program lasts several months, and if collaboration between mental health professionals is not effective, it is troublesome to execute. Finally, the cost of treatment is also an issue. In Greece, this program must be paid for by individuals and is not covered by insurance, but we offer it at a low price to make it available to these people.

The comorbidity of TRSBD and personality disorders presents an awfully imperative clinical issue that can be emerged moreover by the implementation of RECOVERYTRSBDGR. TRSBD and borderline personality disorder, antisocial, schizoid, and histrionic personality disorder is one of the troublesome combinations, according to clinical experience. An antisocial personality disorder doesn't accept the rules of society. These people destroy every interpersonal relationship and are dangerous, showing criminal behavior. A borderline personality disorder shows impulsive, unstable, and auto-destructive behavior. If this impulsive behavior is affected by the positive symptoms, such as hallucinations, this is a very critical situation.

A schizoid prefers lonely activities, and this increases the possibility not coming to group therapy. A histrionic personality seeks attention all the time!

RECOVERYTRSBDGR begins with a restart of pharmacotherapy and a psychoeducation. Afterward, individual cognitive therapy will be implemented, which gives the chance to restructure the schemas of personality disorders and to change dysfunctional behavioral patterns that are also related to personality disorders. Group cognitive behavior therapy and rehabilitation will be implemented in such a way that patients with TRSBD feel capable, step by step, of coping with TRSBD. This enhances the possibility of continuing with group therapy.

That means that antisocial, borderline, histrionic, and schizoid personality disorders have more chances in the context of RECOVERYTRSBDGR to participate in all 140 sessions. The therapeutic relationship that is motivation- and recovery-oriented and activates resources have a positive impact on the above difficult personality disorders.

The following characteristics decrease the plausability of dropping out of RECOVERYTRSBDGR: the presence of two distinct mental health experts—a clinical psychologist and a clinical psychiatrist; open communication about any problem that has arisen within the past, such as non-evidence-based pharmacotherapy and psychotherapies; and the side effects of agents. Furthermore, the treatment of suicidality as a first priority and the implementation of individual and group psychotherapy contribute to upgrading the plausibility of remaining with RECOVERYTRSBDGR and carrying on with the treatment.

The application of motivational interviewing throughout the duration of RECOVERYTRSBDGR can also contribute to the expression of troubles and the center on activity to solve problems. Increasing motivation brings the distance between the state the patient with TRSBD is in and the state to be found closer. The pros and cons of this change need to be discussed in detail. Stagnation will make matters worse. Change will open up new perspectives on life. Increasing motivation can and should occur at each session and sustain retention in treatment. The families of patients with TRSBD are attracted by the increase in motivation and they also participate by contributing to the increase in motivation of the patients. Increasing motivation is, in other words, the key device for proceeding treatment and enduring adversity. It promotes positive thinking and trains a new behavior self-regulation mechanism.

In other words, RECOVERYTRSBDGR takes all the fitting measures to minimize the possibility of dropping out. On the other hand, dropping out could be a part of clinical practice, and we cannot avoid it. Some patients with TRSBD will not take after our vision! Or they require more time to think about their participation. We acknowledge that, and we carry on with other patients who need to participate in our program.

RECOVERYTRSBDGR may be an exceptionally great illustration of the significance of the near and mutual cooperation of clinical psychiatrists and clinical psychologists. This cooperation is characterized by reciprocity, coherence, and respect for the limits of each specialty. Competition, sabotaging the colleague's work, and sending double messages to the patient with TRSBD and the family are unethical and can lead to the dissolution of the therapeutic relationship and treatment. These also create relapses in patients, which are also associated with grief after the loss of another therapeutic relationship with mental health experts.

The finest and most successful programs endure from the human factor or from the plausibility of unsuccessful cooperation between mental health experts. On the off chance that they don't coordinate with each other, no treatment program will work as well as RECOVERYTRSBDGR. So, mental health professionals are responsible for proper cooperation with each other and for the most excellent conceivable implementation of RECOVERYTRSBDGR.

Clinical psychologists and clinical psychiatrists ought to have completed training in cognitive-behavioral psychotherapy, in CR-T (Beck Institute), in metacognitive training (Prof S. Moritz), and in IPT (Prof. V. Roder), so that they can be prepared in our program, the RECOVERYTRSBDGR, and beneath these circumstances they are able to implement it securely.

Evidence-based psychotherapeutic training of mental health experts increases the plausibility of treatment success in RECOVERYTRSBDGR and the arrangement of a long-term therapeutic relationship. Training in cognitive-behavioral psychotherapy creates the foundations for building a structured therapeutic relationship through which mental disorders will be treated with cognitive and behavioral techniques. Typically, the way in which the TRSBD will be treated presupposes clinical involvement with the TRSBD training within cognitive behavioral psychotherapy and further training in structured programs for bipolar disorder and TRSBD, such as our program.

RECOVERYTRSBDGR is a long-term recovery-oriented therapy that gives security, structure, and enhancement in specific areas of the life of patients with TRSBD. It takes a long time to adjust to accept the disorder, the consequences of it, to made changes step by step and to restart life. Patients and their families construct a sustainable, long-term therapeutic relationship with mental health experts.

A long-term therapeutic relationship enhances the motivation for step-by-step improvement in the daily routine under the guidance of a stable therapeutic relationship.

RECOVERYTRSBDGR highlights the advantages of the combination of evidence-based interventions for TRSBD with the probability of a repetition of the therapy in case of a relapse. It is an integrated therapeutic program centered on different levels, such as cognitive dysfunctions, symptoms, and functional outcomes. An integrated program is able to treat, step-by-step, all the resistant dysfunctions, symptoms, and suicidality.

RECOVERYTRSBDGR gives TRSBD patients and their families an understanding of the complications of TRSBD, the consequences of it all these years, why patients feel so weak to manage TRSBD, what measures should be taken by pharmacotherapy in order to avoid polypharmacy and side effects, and which evidence-based psychotherapies should be chosen and why. Patients with TRSBD need more time to learn, to restructure their beliefs regarding their lives, and to adapt to a new reality!

RECOVERYTRSBDGR gives patients with TRSBD and their families hope for a new restart in life. Chronic mental health disorders, such as TRSBD, are confronted with deep grief throughout their lives. RECOVERYTRSBDGR contributes to the change of grief, hopelessness, weakness and loneliness to hope, activity for life, strength, and cohesion with other people, such as mental health experts and family members.

The therapeutic relationship within the setting of RECOVERYTRSBDGR is motivation-, disclosure-, and recovery-oriented. Each session contributes to the improvement of the plausibility of alter. The advantages and disadvantages for every potential of change and progress will be talked about.

Problems and negative emotions will be communicated without stereotypes so that patients with TRSBD and their families can decrease their powerlessness. Grief displays an awfully imperative issue.

The long-term grief with respect to the relapses, the long-term hospitalizations, and the non-adherence to pharmacotherapy and what this means within the past, within the present and within the future will be expressed and analyzed. A difficult situation, such as TRSBD, presents a challenge to reevaluate this unremitting mental health disorder, to alter the entire life and the interpersonal connections, to adjust to a modern reality with reasonable desires, and at least, to be the protagonist of the own difficult situation.

Meaning that patients with TRSBD will take the duty to alter things step by step in life with trust, enactment of resources and adaptability. This status uprgrades their self-esteem and gives them the chance to have a dynamic part in their own lives, which gives them trust for a sustainable future.

The socioeconomic situation in Greece isn't feasible for its citizens. Greece was stood up to with a deep economic crisis from 2008 until today, which influenced the whole nation and especially the health system. The Greek health system doesn't cover the cost of psychotherapeutic sessions.

Patients with TRSBD and other mental health disorders can participate in psychotherapy in the public mental health sectors without financial burden or pay for the psychotherapeutic sessions themselves in the private mental health sector. Patients with TRSBD need another alternative in order to cover the cost of psychotherapeutic sessions. RECOVERYTRSBDGR displays an alternative for these individuals and is adjusted to the needs of patients with TRSBD in Greece.

RECOVERYTRSBDGR offers psychotherapeutic sessions at exceptionally low prices and is adjusted to the troublesome socioeconomic situation of Greece and of TRSBD. Patients with TRSBD are confronted very early with the disorder and they don't have the chance to achieve important life goals. The majority of them take a small amount of social and financial support that doesn't cover the main costs of their lives. This treatment reacts to the social needs of a country, which has not yet come out of the crisis despite what is presented. Patients with chronic mental disorders, such as TRSBD face many economic and social problems and regularly don't have access to modern and specialized psychotherapies.

RECOVERYTRSBDGR will try to fill a gap in Greece and in other countries with respect to the implementation of evidence-based interventions by patients with TRSBD and their families. Greek scientists follow the international evidence-based therapeutic guidelines regarding pharmacotherapy for patients with TRSBD. The absence of an integrated program for patients with TRSBD in Greece and also in other countries, which combines recovery-oriented pharmacotherapy and psychotherapy, presents a reality. Hence, we trust that our program will fill this gap within the scientific community.

Our long-term experiences with TRSBD have highlighted the issues with this disorder all these a long time in Greece. Thus, we have decided to create this recovery-oriented program taking into consideration all the issues of TRSBD: treatment resistance, relapses, hospitalizations, suicidal crises, and non-adherence to the treatments, ECT as a choice and difficulties with that, and huge problems in the interfamilial relationships. A long-term, goal-oriented and recovery-oriented integrative program will be the arrangement to the above-mentioned issues.

It gives sufficient space and time to talk about the negative encounters within the past, to assess the broken choices in pharmacotherapy within the past, to talk openly about all agents, to create a restart in pharmacotherapy, to explain the advantages of every cognitive behavioral psychotherapy and rehabilitation in RECOVERYTRSBDGR, and to implement them step by step.

The family plays an important role in the therapy. 140 sessions in total with the possibility of repetition in case of a relapse present a very motivation-oriented context to prepare the situation for change and transformation in order to achieve a better reintegration into society.

A long-term therapeutic relationship will be developed in order to treat the problems of the past, find solutions in the present, and to be protective umbrella for future crises and relapses.

The maintenance of the therapeutic relationship with the patients with TRSBD and their families even after the completion of RECOVERYTRSBDGR is a very important fact. These patients require time to memorize and hone their skills. The possibility of repeating the program after a relapse also meets the fundamental needs of TRSBD.

Interventions aimed at alleviating the symptoms of bipolar disorder, improving cognitive functions, and functioning from a recovery perspective increase the likelihood of reintegration into society. In this way, the stigma is diminished and the grief is given the opportunity to refine itself and turn into a lasting activity for life.

Resilience is the ability of a person to adapt and cope successfully with negative situations that cause stress [21]. RECOVERYTRSBDGR contributes to resilience because it helps patients with TRSBD and their families accept the disorder, adapt to vulnerabilities and dysfunctions, improve positive beliefs and self-esteem, and recover in the process. This is realized through a mutual, cooperative, and democratic relationship. This procedure of resilience is implemented at the individual and group level; there is also a plausibility to implement couple therapy; and at the very least the program can be repeated, if there is need for that. In other words, resilience is being build up through the combination of individual and group evidence-based pharmacotherapy, and cognitive behavioral psychotherapy and rehabilitation.

Greece has been going through a socioeconomic crisis from 2008 until nowadays. Greece has many structural problems and does not contribute enough funds in the field of health. Our program can be a possibility for evidence-based intervention in combination with the evaluation of its adequacy and efficacy.

Taken together, RECOVERYTRSBDGR presents an outline of evidence-based treatments in TRSBD. The introduction phase tries to register negative experiences. The second phase provides effective evidence-based individual and group psychotherapies. The conclusion is a review of all the changes that have been made. Finally, two monthly follow-ups aim to separate and assess recovery, or subjective recovery. It lasts for 140 sessions. It has advantages and disadvantages. Recovery as an outcome and recovery as a process are important parts of this therapy. Finally, RECOVERYTRSBDGR contributes to the transformation of grief, hopelessness, weakness, and loneliness into hope, action for life, strength, and cohesion with others.

The authors implemented the program over the past 10 months in a pilot study on a sample of five people with TRSBD. It had a positive effect on their lives. Further research studies regarding the efficacy and effectiveness of RECOVERYTRSBDGR (Fig. 4.1) are requested.

4.5 Conclusions

RECOVERYTRSBDGR presents a new proposal for the long-term treatment of TRSBD with advantages and disadvantages. Future studies on the effectiveness and efficacy of this model are required.

Revision Questions
1. Describe the new recovery-oriented pharmacotherapy (RECOVERYTRSBDGR) for TRSBD.
2. Describe the new recovery-oriented psychotherapy (RECOVERYTRSBDGR) for TRSBD.
3. Which is the new element in this new model (RECOVERYTRSBDGR)?
4. What are its advantages and disadvantages?

Competing Interests The authors have no conflicts of interest to declare that are relevant to the content of this chapter.

The authors organize a yearly training on the new recovery-oriented therapy for treatment-resistant bipolar disorder (RECOVERYTRSBDGR) for clinical psychologists, clinical psychiatrists, and cognitive behavioral psychotherapists. For more information, please visit https://www.linkedin.com/in/stavroula-rakitzi-0b512b45/, http://orcid.org/0000-0002-5231-6619 (Stavroula Rakitzi), https://gr.linkedin.com/in/polyxeni-georgila-940b521a7, http://orcid.org/0000-0003-3137-506x (Polyxeni Georgila) or email srakitzi@gmail.com

References

1. Lee JG, Woo YS, Park SW, Seoq DH, Seo MK, Bahk WM. Neuromolecular etiology of bipolar disorder: possible therapeutic targets of mood stabilizers. Clin Psychopharmacol Neurosci. 2022;20(2):228–39. https://doi.org/10.9758/cpn.2022.20.2.228.
2. Zubin J, Spring BJ. Vulnerability – a new view of schizophrenia. J Abnorm Psychol. 1977;86:103–26.
3. Beck AT. Cognitive therapy and the emotional disorders. New York: International University Press; 1976.
4. Palmier-Claus JE, Dodd A, Tai S, Emsley R, Mansell W. Appraisals to affect: testing the integrative cognitive model of bipolar disorder. Br J Clin Psychol. 2016;55(3):225–35. https://doi.org/10.1111/bjc.12081.
5. Donias S, Karastergiou A, Manos N. Standardization of the symptom checklist-90-R rating scale in a Greek population. Psychiatrist. 1991;2(1):42–8.
6. Altman EG, Hedecker D, Peterson JL, Davis M. The Altman self-rating mania scale. Soc Biol Psychiat. 1997;42:948–55.
7. Bech P. Rating scales for psychopathology, health status and quality of life. Berlin: Springer; 1993. p. 325–40.
8. Fountoulakis KN, Iacovides A, Kleanthous S, Samolis S, Gougoulias K, Kaprinis G, Bech P. The Greek translation of the symptoms rating scale for depression and anxiety: preliminary results of the validation study. BMC Psychiatry. 2003;3:21. http://www.biomedcentral.com/1471-244X/3/21.
9. Haddock G, McCarron J, Tarrier N, Faragher EB. Scales to measure dimensions of hallucinations and delusions: the psychotic symptom rating scales (PSYRATS). Psychol Med. 1999;29(4):879–89.
10. World Health Organization. International classification of functioning, disability and health (ICF). Geneva: World Health Organization; 2001.
11. Koumpouros Y, Papageorgiou E, Sakellari E, et al. Adaptation and psychometric properties evaluation of the Greek version of WHODAS 2.0. Pilot application in Greek elderly population. Health Serv Outcome Res Methodol. 2018;18(1):63–74. https://doi.org/10.1007/s10742-017-0176-x.
12. Hancock N, Scanlan JN, Bundy AC, Honey A. Recovery assessment scale –domains & stages (RAS-DS) manual- version 3. Sydney: University of Sydney; 2019.
13. Hancock N, Rakitzi S, Katoudi S. Recovery assessment scale-domains & stages (RAS-DS). The Greek version; 2023.
14. Aster M, Neubauer M, Horn R. Wechsler-Intelligenztest für Erwachsene WIE. Frankfurt: Harcourt Test Services; 2006.
15. Newman CF, Leahy RL, Beck AT, Reilly-Harrington NA, Gyulai L. Bipolar disorder. A cognitive therapy approach. Washington: American Psychological Association; 2003.
16. Beck AT, Grant P, Inverso E, Brinen AP, Perivoliotis D. Recovery oriented cognitive therapy for serious mental health conditions. New York: The Guilford Press; 2021.

17. Haffner P, Quinlivan E, Fiebig J, Sondergeld LM, Strasser ES, Adli M, et al. Improving functional outcome in bipolar disorder: a pilot study on metacognitive training. Clin Psychol Psychother. 2018;25(1):50–8.
18. Miller WR, Rollnick S. Motivational interviewing: preparing people for change. New York: The Guilford Press; 2002.
19. Wu H, Lu L, Qian Y, Jin XH, Yu HR, Du L, Fu XL, ZhuB CHL. The significance of cognitive-behavioral therapy on suicide. An umbrella review. J Affect Disord. 2022;317:142–8. https://doi.org/10.1016/j.jad.2022.08.067.
20. Rakitzi S. Clinical psychology and cognitive behavioral psychotherapy. Recovery in mental health. Cham: Springer; 2023.
21. Shrivastava A, Desousa A. Resilience: a psychobiological construct for psychiatric disorders. In J Psychiatr. 2016;58(1):38–43. https://doi.org/10.4103/0019-5545.174365.

Epilogue

5

Organic and mental health are essential parts that determine human functionality. It is the main core of life. Mental health determines a person's ability to set goals and achieve them, to make realistic plans, to be able to correctly perceive and interpret reality interpersonal relationships, to have good functioning cognitive functions to plan and solve problems.

A huge rate of individuals more promptly acknowledge organic health problems both for themselves and for others. A large rate of individuals moreover have numerous biases against mental health disorders both in themselves and in others. Usually, how the stigma is created. Every individual has the right in life to present health problems and inquire about and offer assistance for them. It is not a shame!

States must bravely finance health systems. A solid health system secures citizens in difficult times, strengthens citizens' sense of security, and at the same time financially supports research on the effectiveness and efficacy of treatments. A treatment is compelling when there is a manual for its application, its objective is obvious and related to research, and research has been conducted on its effectiveness and efficacy. In this way, the treatment gets to be more solid and, at the same time, more available to researchers who need to apply it.

The Greek health system presents numerous structural and financial problems, which have not been settled to date. More specialized interventions are required, particularly within the field of mental health, whose viabiliy will be assesed. Unfortunately, this does not happen systematically in Greece. There is a requirement for more exertion in this course.

The political integration of the European Union can illuminate numerous issues of health systems in Europe if funds are managed better and more of them are contributed in health.

A large percentage of *mental health disorders, bipolar disorder, and TRSBD* in particular belong to the category of resistant disorders. This should concern us from the first session with patients with *affective* disorders. The appearance of a simple

© The Author(s), under exclusive license to Springer Nature
Switzerland AG 2024
S. Rakitzi, P. Georgila, *Treatment-Resistant Bipolar Disorder*,
https://doi.org/10.1007/978-3-031-59001-6_5

depressive episode, which also needs medication, should be the reason to follow it over time and see if it responds positively to the combination of pharmacotherapy and psychotherapy and how it evolves. Does it remain in remission, or are we seeing some behavioral changes, such as hypomanic or manic episodes.

Treatment resistance in mental health disorders has huge rates, according to research studies. This is something that ought to be taken genuinely into consideration. TRSBD presents a distinct category of bipolar disorder. Our encounter with TRSBD led us to think about creating a new, recovery-oriented model. TRSBD needs long-term recovery-oriented and evidence-based pharmacotherapy and psychotherapy.

Mental health experts today have both clinical experience and enough empirical data to make an accurate diagnosis of resistant bipolar disorder as soon as possible. At the same time, many evidence-based psychotherapeutic programs are available for the treatment of bipolar disorder, as presented in Chap. 3 of our book.

What is special about resistant bipolar disorder? Clinical experience in pharmacotherapy and timely application of all effective agents without any delay! The therapeutic relationship between mental health professionals and patients with resistant bipolar disorder will play a crucial role. Initially, dominate suspicion, futility due to successive failed attempts in the past with pharmacotherapy, the desire to die by suicide, and the negotiation to stop the treatment.

Mental health experts are called upon to increase the motivation of patients to try the appropriate agent combinations, which are most effective for them. There will always be a channel of communication for any problem or for any unwanted side effects.

TRSBD is one of the most challenging chronic mental health disorders. Today, we cannot fault the reality that evidence-based pharmacotherapy, psychotherapy, and rehabilitation are not accessible to these people. Research is also continuing and should yield positive results in a few years in terms of pharmacotherapy and psychotherapy.

TRSBD could be a challenge for all of us. We have to be devoted to these individuals in the long term and show profound compassion for them. They have been traumatized in the past by numerous non-evidence-based treatments and have lost faith in mental health experts.

ECT can be effective in bipolar depression. Further research regarding the efficacy of ECT and the impact on cognitive function is needed. The clinical psychiatrist is called upon to exhaust any condition for the most appropriate treatment of patients with TRSBD. ECT can be a possible option for treatment-resistant depression and mania with psychotic features if agents cause severe side effects that lead to severe organic problems, such as cardiological problems. The long-term therapeutic relationship and the adaptation of the proper combination of long-term evidence-based pharmacotherapy and psychotherapy can solve many problems before ECT is selected as a solution, which may not be effective in every patient with TRSBD.

The long-term therapeutic relationship in which the motivation for progressive changes and compliance in pharmacotherapy is expanding needs more time, patience, and adaptability. This road is definitely more difficult because it lasts as long as the patient with TRSBD lives.

So let's give the available modern pharmacotherapy and psychotherapies a chance to be connected. We require more research studies with respect to the effectiveness and efficacy of the combination of evidence-based pharmacotherapy and psychotherapy in a long-term setting. Let us be persistent and flexible with patients with TRSBD and their families, and provide them time to express their negative experiences with treatments in the past.

This will help them understand the significance of legitimate pharmacotherapy in the present without numerous unwanted side effects and the significance of a cooperative therapeutic relationship.

Empirical data regarding the efficacy of pharmacotherapy in TRSBD shows us the way. A combination of antidepressants, mood stabilizers, and antipsychotic agents presents the choices within the setting of pharmacotherapy. After 3 months of pharmacotherapy, mental health experts can continue with recovery-oriented psychotherapy and rehabilitation. This goal-oriented and organized way will decrease the plausibility of relapse and suicidal risk in the future. Research regarding new agents for bipolar disorder and TRSBD is in process, and we expect new agents and possibly genetic therapies.

The next step for mental health professionals is to increase the motivation to participate in psychotherapeutic programs, which are implemented over a long period of time and aim at interventions at many levels with the main goal of generalized improvement of functioning. The more persistent the mental disorder, the more time needed for psychotherapy.

Long-term psychotherapy has the advantage of continuously assessing progress and difficulties in coping with the dysfunctions that result from bipolar disorder. It also reduces the likelihood of frequent hospitalizations in the depressive or manic phase.

Excellent psychotherapies are available to us today. What we need to test in the future is the combination of various effective treatments with each other, as in pharmacotherapy, and what impact this has on the lives of patients with bipolar and resistant bipolar disorder. RECOVERYTRSBDGR includes all the above components.

Long-term treatment that centers on recovery will help them recapture certainty in their treatment. Long-term outpatient treatment focused on recovery will help them discover new meaning in life, avoid unnecessary hospitalizations, claim all rights to better reintegrate into society, and become protagonists in their own lives in the context of recovery.

RECOVERYTRSBDGR, a new ambulant program focused on recovery, is leading the way. It consists of three phases and gradually sets the scene for a modern restart of pharmacotherapy and psychotherapy. Cognitive, metacognitive, and recovery perspectives play an important role within the structure of the therapy.

Research regarding new agents for bipolar disorder and TRSBD is in process, and we expect new medications and possibly genetic therapies in the future. *Genetic therapies will eliminate the root of this disorder. On the other hand, it is very difficult to find an exact genetic therapy that will root out the treatment-resistant depressive and manic-hypomanic symptoms as well as the treatment-resistant cognitive dysfunction.*

Until this day comes, we have to be patient and carry on with the available long-term evidence-based interventions for patients with TRSBD. RECOVERYTRSBDGR displays an opportunity in that direction and can also support patients with TRSBD in case of the existence of genetic therapies.

We hope that RECOVERYTRSBDGR will inspire us and other colleagues to execute it more systematically and evaluate its effectiveness and efficiency.

Patients with TRSBD and their families need more time to learn, adapt to challenges, and find their own rhythm in life within the context of evidence-based treatments.

It is conceivable to battle against TRSBD and learn to cope without getting disorganized, without strong suicidal risk, and without stigma. The new meaning of life is to become a good master of your own problems!

Science has given us the opportunity to find new dimensions in modern therapies, and we ought to be grateful for that. We are even more thankful to our patients because developing a therapy would not be conceivable without the presence and contributions of people with TRSBD and their families.

Eventually, transforming weak, suspicious, suicidal, and socially isolated patients with TRSBD into active people, open to new life experiences, with new meaning to their lives and integrating into society by claiming all their rights, is one of the most prominent involvements for all mental health experts.

Polypharmacy, side effects due to polypharmacy, and the implementation of non-evidence-based treatments display traumatic experiences for patients with TRSBD. As mental health experts, we are obliged to have the appropriate training and clinical experience as clinical psychologists, clinical psychiatrists, and cognitive behavioral psychotherapists with patients with TRSBD and with evidence-based treatments.

We should be able to educate them to recognize some very dangerous aspects: Are the criteria for polypharmacy and non-evidence-based treatments by previous mental health experts evidence-based? Can these parameters lead to suicide? Yes!

Many patients with TRSBD have been confronted with traumas during their lives. Physical, sexual, and psychological abuse appears very often by these individuals. When polypharmacy and non-evidence-based psychotherapies are added to this terrible repertoire of life events, the possibility of relapse and disorganization is very big! This special category of patients with TRSBD deserves our devotion and respect.

Our book could be a journey to evidence-based treatments for patients with TRSBD and their families. It is written in a simple way that is reasonable for non-experts. Hence, we want to help these people know the truth about TRSBD, the problems that are related to it, the evidence-based interventions that are available, how to avoid malpractice by mental health experts, and what are their human rights regarding access to recovery-oriented treatments.

Governments in all over the world ought to fund psychotherapy for mental health disorders through insurances.

The Greek insurance system doesn't cover the cost of psychotherapy, and there is no intention toward such an objective, which is exceptionally dangerous and disappointing. Greek psychiatric departments in clinics, ambulant settings in the public and private sectors, and private practices in Greece should be evaluated through Greek governments and Greek scientific associations regarding the efficacy of evidence-based treatments. RECOVERYTRSBDGR can fill this gap in Greece and in other countries. GREECE does not offer enough financial support for research in mental health.

RECOVERYTRSBDGR protects patients with TRSBD from multiple traumas, such as polypharmacy, non-evidence-based psychotherapy, and abusive behaviors of mental health experts. Patients know which interventions are going to be implemented, in what order, and which therapeutic objectives are planned to be accomplished with every intervention. Two mental health experts are available during the whole process and are obliged to work professionally. Abusive behaviors have no place in our recovery program.

The introduction phase tries to enlist negative experiences and contribute to a new restart within the setting of evidence-based treatments. The second phase provides viable evidence-based individual and group psychotherapies. The conclusion is a review of all the changes that have been made. At long last, 2 monthly follow-ups aim to separate and assess recovery or subjective recovery. Psychiatric treatment is the main therapy and takes place once a month. Individual and group psychotherapy within the framework of cognitive-behavioral psychotherapy and rehabilitation is an adjunct therapy to pharmacotherapy. A psychological assessment will be given pre-intervention, post-intervention, and at 6-month follow-up (recovery as an outcome).

RECOVERYTRSGR keeps going with 140 sessions and educates individuals with TRSBD and their families how to manage bipolar disorder, TRSBD, and suicidal risk, improving cognitive functions and symptoms, recovery, and functional outcome results. This ambulatory setting minimizes the probability of hospitalization and increments the probability of living within the community in the context of social reintegration centered on recovery.

RECOVERYTRSBDGR has many advantages. Specific evidence-based psychiatric and psychotherapeutic treatments are being offered in one program. Long-term implementation gives the mental health experts a huge chance to improve the resistant cognitive dysfunctions, the depressive and manic symptoms, and the functional outcome, and to see the advance of these improvements over the time. A therapeutic relationship with these people is built through our program. They have the right to express their difficulties with the treatment, to declare more help from the experts, and to set their claim limits, in case something is not right for them. Mental health experts are there to teach patients with TRSBD making a wonderful scientific journey.

In other words, RECOVERYTRSBDGR follows democratic conditions and rejects each form of abuse by mental health experts to patients with TRSBD and their families.

The disadvantages of RECOVERYTRSBDGR can be the long-term implementation and the numerous therapies that are available. Patients with TRSBD experience relapses, hospitalizations, suicidal crisis, and many problems with the family. They lost their hope to do anything! If a long-term commitment is proposed, this can be very difficult for them after many failures in the therapy. RECOVERYTRSBDGR offers an opportunity to make a restart with the pharmacotherapy and to speak openly about all the problems and stereotypes regarding pharmacotherapy and psychotherapy. Patients with TRSBD should have enough time and space to decide whether they are going to participate in it or not. Our clinical experience showed us that individuals have more possibility to come if they know all the truth about their mental health disorder and the possible therapies.

RECOVERYTRSBDGR gives the opportunity to construct step by step a secure and steady therapeutic relationship that gives openings to talking straightforwardly around issues with TRSBD with past non-evidence-based treatments, with limits in the context of the therapeutic relationship, and to give patients with TRSBD enough time and space to test the changes and to adjust them step by step on every day routine. The therapeutic relationship within the setting of RECOVERYTRSBDGR is motivation-oriented, goal-oriented with certain limits, and actuates the appropriate resources by patients with TRSBD in order to carry on with the recovery as a process.

This therapeutic relationship contributes to the mindfulness of the issue via systematic psycho-education and to the alteration of the most issues, such as symptoms, cognitive dysfunctions, and dysfunctional thoughts and schemas that have a negative impact on quality of life and functional outcomes. Finally, this relationship transforms the grief regarding TRSBD into action for life.

Grief presents a tremendous issue. Patients with TRSBD and their families spend many years grieving the existence of the disorder. The five stages of grief, shock, denial, anger, depression, and acceptance-reboot show a better way to manage this burden and its consequences. Patients manifest to express their grief with depressive and manic symptoms and family members with chronic depression. Our first contact with them always has almost the same characteristics: relapses, hospitalizations that did not go well, anger, and despair. We become listeners to this pain and grief. We must, before starting any intervention, give space and time for this burden to be expressed.

Grief management has advantages and disadvantages. Disadvantages focus on the fact that, in the short-term, depression may occur and there may be poor adherence to treatment. The advantages long-term are greater. This emotional burden has been given a chance to express itself and not continually lead to relapse. The method of acknowledgment and restart makes a difference within the long term to better manage the disorder and to take individual responsibility for mental health enhancement.

Grief management also helps better manage the stigma of the mental health disorders. The burden encompassing the mental health disorder is communicated and, at the same time, given the opportunity to be set within the person's memory and soul in a setting that will not disturb the person's everyday life.

In this way, the individuals acknowledges himself/herself and his or her disorder way better, and does not feel embarrassed or hopeless, does not isolate himself/herself, and looks for ways to live with this disorder. In this manner, the stigma against the disorder is diminished. RECOVERYTRSBDGR is an activity for life and centers on step-by-step enhancement on numerous levels, such as cognitive, emotional, and behavioral level, and this method contributes to a better coping with the disorder and its grief as well as with the stigma with respect to TRSBD.

RECOVERYTRSBDGR can moreover offer assistance patients with TRSBD and severe personality disorders. If patients learn to manage with TRSBD and to restructure schemas that are associated with the psychopathology, this would also have a positive impact on their personality disorder. CBTp and CR-T reduce the burden of dysfunctional schemas, which are also associated with personality disorders. Cognitive restructuring, behavior modification, and social skills that are included in RECOVERYTRSBDGR are also successful for the treatment of personality disorders.

Additionally, the long-term implementation of our treatment in 140 sessions gives us enough space and time to center indirectly on schemas and behaviors that are related with personality disorders. On the other hand, RECOVERYTRSBDGR has as a first priority the treatment of TRSBD but can intervene indirectly on the level of personality disorders. It is also known and clear from clinical practice that when TRSBD is being treated well, this has a positive impact on the level of dysfunction in personality.

When patients with TRSBD are confronted with traumas, such as physical, sexual and psychological abuse, it is recommended to work very carefully with traumas, implementing cognitive restructuring of thoughts and beliefs and not exposure to trauma. Exposure can lead to a relapse, specifically to a depressive or manic episode with a suicidal crisis and hospitalization.

A balance between benefits and costs ought to continuously be our main orientation when choosing the best conceivable interventions for TRSBD in cases of trauma. The worst scenario, according to our clinical practice, is the abuse of patients with TRSBD by parents or family members, and by mental health experts.

A mental health expert, whom the patient with TRSBD trusted, built a therapeutic relationship with him and tried through it to alter things and improve his quality of life. He abused his trust and abused him/her. It is the worst form of abuse of power. Scientific companies are called upon to empower patients to report incidents of violence and to support them in addressing the prosecutorial and judicial authorities.

The trauma of abuse always remains deeply established within the depressive, manic-hypomanic, and psychotic symptoms. It takes a long time to make it manageable as well as a new restart with it.

Let's respect the chronicity of TRSBD and its burden. Let's regard the fact that it is the most troublesome chronic mental disorder with a high plausibility of suicide. Let us regard the reality that some of our fellow citizens develop, during their lifetime, a chronic mental disorder with a high rate of disability and a high hazard of suicide.

The quality of our democracy is measured by how well it can expand a security net to our vulnerable fellow citizens, how well it appears to be the way of protecting them from conceivable mishandling of power, and the opportunities it gives them to restore and reintegrate into society.

The European Union is requesting to assess all its members who received funds to strengthen mental health services. The questions that arise are the following: How much money did each country get, and where was it channeled? Are evidence-based interventions implemented and is their effectiveness evaluated? Are there safeguards against abuse of power, and how are they actualized?

The European Union must be the matrix of democracy, which is able to protect itself without the citizen having to form reports about whether our vulnerable fellow citizens, such as patients with TRSBD, are ensured by the member states. Particularly in Greece, are evidence-based interventions being implemented in mental health services (public and private sector), is polypharmacy avoided in patients with TRSBD, under which conditions is ECT applied by patients with TRSBD?

Treatment discontinuation is a gigantic problem in TRSBD. RECOVERYTRSBDGR has the following characteristics, which diminish the possibility of treatment interference: the cohesive collaboration of two diverse mental health experts—a clinical psychologist and a clinical psychiatrist; an honest communication almost any issue, such as non-evidence-based pharmacotherapy and psychotherapies;

and the side effects of agents. Moreover, the treatment of suicidal risk as a first priority and the implementation of individual and group psychotherapy enhance the motivation for remaining at RECOVERYTRSBDGR. The application of motivational interviewing throughout the duration of RECOVERYTRSBDGR also enhances the motivation for the therapy.

On the other hand, dropping out is a part of clinical practice, and we cannot avoid it. Some patients with TRSBD will not follow our vision! Or they require more time to think about their cooperation.

RECOVERYTRSBDGR can be depicted as an individual who strolls within the sea and observes the state of the sea well. If she is stormy, the person won't come in and wait doing other things. At the same time, the individual will try to reduce the stress from the stormy sea, improve the mood with other activities, and not be possessed by the grandiosity that the person will succeed in entering the stormy sea. The individual will enter the sea when it is calm and enjoy it. This way, the person will be able to manage the sea in realistic and feasible contexts.

The calm sea offers peace and security. These conditions will help in a better management of everyday life, in the better assertion of the rights of the person, as well as in better protection from abuse and professional unethical behavior.

The calm sea helps to make more realistic decisions and strengthens optimism for the future. This leads to the improvement of TRSBD with limits, rules, and possibilities for development through the activation of resources. The above conditions are the best conditions for dealing with any incidents of patient abuse.

Patients with TRSBD are enabled through treatment and know how to recognize between evidence-based interventions and non-evidence-based treatments. RECOVERYTRSBDGR shows a structured and transparent psychotherapeutic path to improve functional outcomes and quality of life. Structure and transparency engage problem-solving as well as resistance to any form of abuse by mental health professionals.

RECOVERYTRSBDGR displays the importance of the close and mutual cooperation of clinical psychiatrists and clinical psychologists that is characterized by reciprocity, coherence, and respect. Competition, sabotaging the colleague's work, and sending double messages to the patient with TRSBD and the family are unethical and can lead to the dissolution of the therapeutic relationship and treatment. Competition and sabotage have no place in the face of the psychological and emotional burden of TRSBD. The value and dignity of human life are far more important than the competition and selfishness among mental health experts.

The essential prerequisite for the application of the RECOVERYTRSBDGR by clinical psychologists and clinical psychiatrists is a completed training in cognitive-behavioral psychotherapy, in CR-T (Beck Institute), in metacognitive training (Prof S. Moritz), and in IPT (Prof. V. Roder), so that they can be trained afterward by us in our program-the RECOVERYTRSBDGR. Evidence-based psychotherapeutic training of mental health experts increases the possibility of treatment success in RECOVERYTRSBDGR.

Patients with TRSBD and their families, who took part in the pilot group of RECOVERYTRSBDGR, have expressed the following impressions:

(A) 140 sessions! It was the first time I participated in so many sessions. I was anxious and curious at the beginning because I had negative experiences with mental health experts in the past. At the end of the treatment, I had the feeling that I know better, I accepted, and I can control my serious mental health disorder. It was worth it.

(B) I have improved my concentration, my depressive symptoms, and my sleep and I understand better the significance of adherence to pharmacotherapy. I can achieve now new goals in my life.

(C) RECOVERYTRSBDGR has helped me to understand the negative effects of TRSBD in my life, how psychotherapy works, and that I am also responsible for my mental health each day. I hope that the Greek insurance system will cover the cost of this psychotherapy in the future.

(D) The combination of individual and group therapy is very interesting. My family shows more empathy for me. The verbal and psychological abuse toward me has been disrupted

(E) I have learned that there are numerous accessible treatments for TRSBD. I fight in 140 sessions to improve my mental health. It is like a marathon. I run also the real marathon in Athens! I have made new friends, who have the same issue as me. Transparency, cohesion, and goal-oriented behavior helped me to build a new relationship with TRSBD and with my family.

(F) I feel more secure as the mother of a son with TRSBD to manage this serious mental health disorder. We fight together every day with dignity, love and cohesion.

(G) As father of a daughter who suffers from TRSBD I would like the following comments: I spend many hours with my daughter in psychiatric departments trying to fix the suicidality. It is terrible for me to hear my child say that death is the only perspective for her. I hope that new therapies will come in the next few years in order to fix TRSBD better. RECOVERYTRSBDGR has taught us the following: my child suffers from TRSBD, there are specific agents which are effective for it; I accepted this mental health disorder better; and my daughter manage better her depressive and manic symptoms as well as her suicidality. She tries now to finish her studies; the future will be better!

(H) The bipolar disorder of my brother was a nightmare for me. I didn't know how to behave the next day and what awaited me. I was physical and psychological abused from my brother in his manic phase. RECOVERYTRSBDGR helped me to understand what TRSBD is, how can I improve my communication with my brother and how can I set my limits toward him. I put limits on abuse.

(I) My grief for TRSBD is what I can describe as a maze. I was lost in it for 10 years. Relapses, hospitalizations and suicidality. My child lost, and so am I with him. We heard about the new treatment, and it opened a door. I could see my child getting better, and I was slowly coming out of my grief.

(J) The stigma of mental illness has led to isolation, a lack of hope for a potentially effective treatment, and isolation from the health system and mental health professionals. But the isolation led to many hospitalizations for my child with depressive and manic episodes. Stigma has led us to destruction. Participating in RECOVERYTRSBDGR helped us de-stigmatize TRSBD and learn to manage it.

A patient who participated in RECOVERYTRSBDGR has decided to write a letter to our recovery-oriented therapy:

Dear RECOVERYTRSBDGR,

I wanted to die by suicide for many years. I have gone to numerous mental health experts who have prescribed many medications. I slept all day. I was very desperate regarding my life and daily routine. I attempted to find a job, without success.

A friend of mine who suffers from TRSBD has referred me to Dr. Georgila and Dr. Rakitzi. I met them in five sessions to arrange to clarify how RECOVERYTRSBDGR can help me. I decided to start with this therapy.

I have learned the problems of TRSBD, why I took so numerous medications from past psychiatrists, and why clozapine and lithium helped me. I suffer from

TRSBD and the balance regarding my pharmacotherapy depends on my adherence. I take my agents every day because I know why! Cognitive-behavioral psychotherapy and metacognitive therapy had helped me manage my anxiety, my depression, and my hallucinations. I recognize my depressive and manic phases and I contact with Dr. Georgila and Dr. Rakitzi if something changes for me. I control my psychopathology better. I have improved my relationship with my family. We spend a lot of time together without verbal abuse. I was attacked by my family in the past with verbal abuse. Dr. Rakitzi and Dr. Georgila have trained us to communicate with each other without abuse. I am not the bipolar disorder; this is my disorder. So they have to respect that! I fight every day against TRSBD. There's always a way to manage the negative consequences of a mental health disorder, and that's what I have learned with RECOVERYTRSBDGR.

The mother of the patient who participated on RECOVERYTRSBDGR has chosen, moreover, to type in a letter to our recovery-oriented therapy:

Dear RECOVERYTRSBDGR,

Depression, weakness, and no hope for the future. These words show my feelings as psychiatrists have announced the diagnosis of bipolar disorder by my son. I was in a severe depression for many years. I was also diagnosed with bipolar disorder but not a TRSBD.

My son took a lot of medications and couldn't stay alone at home. He was depressed for many months during the year, slept a lot of hours, and wanted to die by suicide. Manic phases came after depression. He couldn't sleep, was very aggressive, spent a lot of money, and heard voices. I didn't trust mental health experts anymore.

A friend of my son has referred us to Dr. Georgila and Dr. Rakitzi. I didn't need to meet new mental health experts! My son wanted it a lot!

140 sessions! So many! This therapy is offered at low prices, and therefore I could finance it. I communicate better with my son. We spend more time together, helping him to come to his objectives. My depression has decreased. My son learned that he suffers from a subcategory of bipolar disorder, the TRSBD.

He found a new meaning in his life. It is clear for us that polypharmacy isn't essential, that side effects bring more problems, and that we have the right to fight against malpractice.

TRSBD can be coped with, like other health and mental health problems. Participation in a long-term therapeutic program is the key to success. I am very proud of my son and of my family that we have achieved cohesion and a restart in our lives!

A patient who participated in RECOVERYTRSBDGR wrote the following letter:

Dear RECOVERYTRSBDGR,

My father abandoned me when I was 15 years old. I grew up with my mother and grandmother. I had my first major depressive episode at 18 and 10 months after my first manic episode with psychotic features. I was hospitalized. We lived for many years in isolation, we felt stigmatized and an immense shame. I stopped the medication because I saw no point in continuing it. I changed many doctors. We lived isolated in our house with immense shame.

I decided to participate in this treatment because I wanted to try something different. The last chance! Structured intervention began. I learned to manage the depressive and manic symptoms as well as the thoughts associated with them.

A father of a young girl who participated in RECOVERYTRSBDGR has written a letter to our recovery-oriented therapy:

Dear RECOVERYTRSBDGR,

I have the opportunity to participate in RECOVERYTRSBDGR on the occasion of my daughter's participation. She is 28 years old and was diagnosed with bipolar disorder 3 years ago. Pharmacotherapy was not effective according to her and therefore discontinued it. She was hospitalized two times with a manic episode with psychotic features. She had a monthly psychiatric treatment the last 12 months. The psychiatrist didn't propose any psychotherapy.

A friend of my daughter told us about RECOVERYTRSBDGR. The long-term implementation of a therapy was comforting to me. My daughter would have a new family and two female therapists.

This was very important because my wife died after fighting 3 years with the cancer. Six months later my daughter had her first manic episode.

A patient who participated in RECOVERYTRSBDGR but dropped out has chosen to compose a letter to our recovery-oriented therapy:

Dear RECOVERYTRSBDGR,

My life is exceptionally difficult with bipolar disorder. I was hospitalized many times and I have changed many psychiatrists. I have heard about RECOVERYTRSBDGR from another patient.

I visited Dr. Georgila and Dr. Rakitzi and I decided to participate in this therapy. 140 sessions! I thought that i would not be able to do all these 140 sessions! Dr. Georgila clarified to me that we will begin with major changes in my pharmacotherapy, which could help the RECOVERYTRSBDGR. Dr. Georgila clarified TRSBD for me.

After 12 years of bipolar disorder, I learned what TRSBD is! This information helped me understand how troublesome my mental health disorder is.

I live in a family with many problems. My father suffers from schizophrenia, my mother from bipolar disorder, and my sister has a substance abuse disorder. We are very isolated, and we all have many agents. I didn't have any support from them to participate in RECOVERYTRSBD. I felt exhausted by this family. I participate in the first 20 sessions of the RECOVERYTRSBDGR. I couldn't carry on.

Dr. Rakitzi and Dr. Georgila have proposed that I carry on with an intensive psychiatric treatment twice monthly by Dr. Georgila. I try to find a new meaning in my life by finding a new job, and when I am ready, I can try once again with the RECOVERYTRSBDGR.

I know exactly now what TRSBD means, and if I follow every day with discipline my pharmacotherapy, I would be able to work a part-time job.

A patient with bipolar disorder and borderline personality disorder has written a letter to RECOVERYTRSBDGR.

Dear RECOVERYTRSBDGR,

I was hospitalized in many psychiatric departments in Athens. I have been treated by many directors of psychiatric departments as well as by many psychiatrists and many psychologists in private practice.

I had many side effects from the polypharmacy and many health problems. I had many suicidal plans and I wanted to die by suicide. I felt depressed most of the year, and for 4 months a year I was strong, impulsive, and very excited regarding my life. I had two personalities!

Dr. Rakitzi referred me to Dr. Georgila, who treats me monthly. I am treated know with clozapine and lithium, and Dr. Georgila explained that I suffer from TRSBD, which is why I have two different phases during the year. It is not my personality but my affective disorder. Dr. Georgila proposed me to participate in RECOVERYTRSBDGR, which I accepted it.

140 sessions! It was the first time that I participated in such structured and transparent psychotherapy. My parents and my husband participate in psycho-education and learned to show more empathy toward me. The combination of my affective disorder and my personality disorder leads to all these problems, and not my two personalities. I am not dangerous or strange.

The combination of individual and group therapy helped me to better manage my cognitive distortions, which are associated with my thoughts. This helped me to manage my depression and mania and to accept the impulsiveness of my personality. I am the mother of a boy and a girl, and I want to be strong enough in the future to support them.

I met other people with the same problems. I am not alone; we are a big family. It is a petty that I have spent my young years in psychiatric departments with many hospitalizations because nobody could explain to me what TRSBD is. I deserve a better treatment as a human being, and I will not allow any expert in the future to treat me like an experiment in mental health disorders. As we explained, recovery is in process. Every day I try to improve myself and to be strong as a mother for my lovely children.

Patients with mental health disorders in Greece deserve more respect and access to evidence-based treatments in clinical psychiatry and clinical psychology.

The sister of a patient who participated in RECOVERYTRSBDGR gave the following feedback:

Dear RECOVERYTRSBDGR,

My brother suffers from treatment-resistant bipolar I disorder. He was hospitalized many times the last 3 years. It was very difficult to find a way to cope with it. I was afraid of my brother. He was very aggressive during the manic phases and I was unfortunately many times physical and psychological abused from my brother.

Dr. Rakitzi and Dr. Georgila proposed me to participate in the psycho-education phase of this program. I reject it but they persuaded me to be part of this restart in our family. I have understand what bipolar I disorder is and what resistant bipolar I disorder is. It was the first time that I heard about what treatment-resistant bipolar disorder is.

The abusive behavior of my brother was the consequence of a resistant manic episode with grandiosity thoughts.

They refer me to a cognitive behavioral psychotherapist to work my depression, my grief and a possible PTSD.

I feel better now that I can understand what is going on with my brother. We spend time together during the week without anxiety and panic!

Dear RECOVERYTRSBDGR,

I am a grandmother raising her grandson, 22 years old, My grandson has bipolar disorder and lives with me because his parents died by suicide when he was 13 years old. They themselves suffered from bipolar disorder. I have visited all the hospitals in Athens. All the doctors were trying to convince him that medication is the main treatment.

He was taking them for a month, he was fine but he was complaining about being sedated, which led to bad compliance. He didn't sleep, fighted with me, and abused me.

A doctor recommended RECOVERYTRSBDGR. I promised my grandson that he will not be hospitalized again, but we will go to treatment together.

We were informed about the resistant bipolar disorder. I understood why there was a problem with the pharmacotherapy. Dr. Georgila discussed openly all the issues with him and put him on agents, which helps him sleep well but is active during the day. He has thoughts that he could do nothing in his life. But it's not like that after all.

He learned to process his negative thoughts, entered a program of mood-enhancing activities and continues his studies. We have a great time together and he respects me. He met other young people who have the same problem and made new friends.

He is very sad due to many hospitalizations in the past and afraid for the future. But he found a new family and feels safe. His own effort contributed to the fact that he was not hospitalized again.

The father and mother of a 25 year old wrote the following letter:

Dear RECOVERYTRSBDGR,

We have been living a nightmare for 8 years. We spend a lot of time in the psychiatric departments of hospitals every 2 months. Our son was not taking his agents and thought he would solve the problems on his own. He had many manic episodes with psychotic elements. We learned about this new treatment. We suggested our son go and try psychotherapy for his anxiety. He accepted and that's how our journey with RECOVERYTRSBDGR began. Mrs. Georgila did several sessions with him to explain the agents in detail and to feel safe starting them. Mrs. Rakitzi also did many sessions with psycho-education and increasing motivation.

His participation in the program ended and he is now doing couple therapy with his girlfriend to improve the relationship. We celebrate every day and have finally found a way to move into life action and leave behind our grief and stigma, which had plunged us into, despair and a permanent fear of our own death and our own son's death.

The parents of a 30-year-old woman who did not continue RECOVERYTRSBDGR wrote the following letter:

Dear RECOVERYTRSBDGR,

The first communication with Dr. Georgila and Dr. Rakitzi gave us hope! We had been tired for the past 8 years with bipolar I disorder and many relapses. Our daughter was very tired and could not find any meaning in her life!

We did the psycho-education together with our daughter, who had already started her new psychiatric treatment in the last two months. They explained to us what resistant bipolar disorder is! That was a relief.

Our daughter continued with her individual therapy and psychiatric follow-up, but was found to be a chronic substance abuser. Ms. Georgila told us that RECOVERYTRSBDGR should temporarily stop and the therapy should focus on substance abuse. Then she could continue in RECOVERYTRSBDGR. When the substance abuse problem was revealed, it was easier to understand why our daughter was relapsing! We felt a lot of guilt about not understanding anything. Our daughter has been in the psychiatric department for substance abuse for a long time. She promised us that she will continue with RECOVERYTRSBDGR.

The impressions of our patients with TRSBD and the briefs to RECOVERYTRSBDGR display the recovery in process through our program.

It is an honor for us to have met all these people who favored our RECOVERYTRSBDGR. It is an honor for us to offer a recovery-oriented therapy.

Research studies regarding the effectiveness and efficacy of our therapy are in demand.

The combination of clinical implementation and research helps us to realize the needs of our patients and their families and the appropriate recovery-oriented programs for them.

The following conclusions can be drawn from these briefs regarding RECOVERYTRSBDGR:

Bipolar disorder and TRSBD can be under diagnosed or misdiagnosed. Mental health experts need time to give such as a diagnosis and should follow all the evidence-based criteria for the diagnostic procedure, the pharmacotherapy and psychotherapy.

It is exceptionally important to clarify transparently what TRSBD is and why it is a particulate category in bipolar disorder.

Pharmacotherapy in TRSBD is the main therapy and ought to be adjusted appropriately before beginning with cognitive-behavioral therapy and rehabilitation.

Psycho-education can help the family understand the challenges of TRSBD and can offer an alternative way of communication without verbal abuse.

The combination of individual and group therapy in RECOVERYTRSBDGR provides many ways to manage resistant cognitive dysfunctions, depressive and manic symptoms, as well as suicidality. This improves functional outcome and quality of life.

The cognitive, metacognitive, and recovery perspectives show the leading response to the treatment of TRSBD!

The coexistence of TRSBD and personality disorders presents a big challenge during the therapy. The borderline personality disorder is a special category. When a dual diagnosis of TRSBD and borderline personality disorder is being given, it is very important in the context of RECOVERYTRSBDGR to learn to cope with TRSBD and then to see the impact of it on the personality disorder.

The combination of evidence-based treatments in RECOVERYTRSBDGR can support the cope with the problems of borderline personality disorder.

If patients with TRSBD have comorbid substance abuse disorders, it is recommended to treat substance abuse and to ensure adherence to pharmacotherapy and afterward to continue with RECOVERYTRSBDGR.

RECOVERYTRSBDGR prevents abuse between the family members and educates people to be assertive toward numerous forms of abuse and malpractice by mental health experts and in life generally.

RECOVERYTRSBDGR educates patients to cope with TRSBD, and this is a pattern for dealing with other resistant problems in life, such as health and social problems.

RECOVERYTRSBDGR displays a democratic therapy, which protects the rights and needs of patients with TRSBD and their families.

Bipolar disorder and TRSBD display chronic mental health disorders. Patients and their families learn to manage them for their whole lives. A coexistence with a chronic mental health disorder needs long-term professional treatment and evidence-based therapy. The activation of the appropriate resources contributes to a new and positive way of dealing with a severe mental health disorder.

RECOVERYTRSBDGR is able to activate these resources and help people restart their lives in a setting with reasonable objectives.

Mental health experts who choose to work with chronic mental health disorders need good training and education, clinical experience, and the ability to take care of themselves.

An education in clinical psychiatry, in clinical psychology, in cognitive behavioral psychotherapy, huge clinical experience with patients with bipolar disorder and TRSBD, and lifelong training in programs and psychotherapies for patients withbipolardisorderarethesuitableconditionstoimplementRECOVERYTRSBDGR.

RECOVERYTRSBDGR combines famous evidence-based interventions with each other. Pharmacotherapy is the principal therapy and is combined with evidence-based cognitive behavioral therapy and rehabilitation. Psycho-education ought to be combined contributes to increased awareness and insight toward bipolar disorder.

CBT contributes to a better coping with depressive, manic, and hypomanic symptoms, which reduces distress from them, and it also contributes to the improvement of anxiety and quality of life. The cognitive restructuring of various schemata, such as the vulnerability, weakness, and grandiosity schemas, presents a key component in this treatment.

CT-R presents the newest development of the Beck Group in the USA for serious mental health disorders. CT-R focuses on activating positive beliefs and actions in the context of TRSBD, which leads to resilience and recovery. MCT, a metacognitive intervention, presents a short-term intervention. It is a combination of CBT and rehabilitation, and it can be implemented in a group setting.

Psycho-education improves the family dynamic, reduces critical comments or emotional over-involvement of members toward people with TRSBD, improves the communication between them, and rebuilds the dysfunctional schema of the family members.

It is recommended to offer couple therapy after the end of RECOVERYTRSBDGR. Integrative Behavioral Couple Therapy focuses on three strategies in therapy: the affective change enhancing empathy, the cognitive change enhancing a new point of view of the problem, and the behavioral change enhancing new coping with the problem and can be implemented.

Improvement in bipolar disorder after treatment can free up the potential for a relationship to continue. The person with TRSBD can better regulate their thinking and mood after RECOVERYTRSBDGR. This also has an impact on communication and cooperation within the relationship.

Thus, couples therapy can improve the atmosphere in the relationship with more days of caring and the restructuring of negative beliefs about the relationship. It can also reduce the stigma of TRSBD in the relationship.

The benefits of couple therapy are continued relationship recovery and improvement, increased likelihood of maintaining the marriage and relationship, and destigmatization of TRSBD within the relationship. The disadvantages of couple therapy include possible fatigue from long-term psychotherapy. There is no other way. Action for life against stigma, isolation, fear of death, suicidal risk, and hopelessness is implemented through long-term pharmacotherapy and psychotherapy.

The combination of individual and group therapy with different contents, that is, the individual alone with cognitive behavioral therapy and recovery therapy which reinforces positive beliefs, then the patient in metacognitive training with other patients with TRSBD. Psycho-education presents also a very interesting group context, in which awareness is being achieved. Finally, there is the recommendation for the application of couple therapy after the end of RECOVERYTRSBDGR.

In other words, patients with TRSBD participate in numerous therapeutic contexts building therapeutic relationships with mental health experts in individual and group settings. This increases awareness of the disorder by better understanding the importance of stable pharmacotherapy. It also enhances communication, flexibility, and empathy in human relationships. Others present model learning and inspire change.

All this effort gives a new meaning to life: the action for improvement and a better quality of life. So in this way, chronic suicidality can be better treated.

Working with chronic mental health disorders means that experts ought to activate their own resources and find time to do other things, such as entertainment, traveling, spending time with family and friends, and getting to know new cultures. A great psycho-hygiene activates more motivation in TRSBD therapy, decreases anxiety, and increases the effectiveness of mental health experts.

Bipolar disorder and TRSBD are so universal. So it is exceptionally imperative to get to know other cultures as well. So it will be awesome when RECOVERYTRSBDGR is implemented in many nations around the world.

Patients with bipolar disorder and TRSBD suffer from a long-term grief. Why am I sick? It's my fault? Are bad relationships in the family to blame? I spent so many years with hospitalizations, suicide attempts, substance abuse, and social isolation. Why me?

Grief therapy presents a key part of psychotherapy for chronic mental health disorders, such as bipolar disorder. Psycho-education increases awareness. Patients must go through all the phases of Grief: shock, anger, denial, depression, acceptance, and reboot or restart. Mental health experts should be very careful with grief because it can be expressed through a rapid switch off between mania and depression or rapid mood fluctuations.

Unfortunately, we cannot change the past or the dysfunction of neurotransmitters. The difficult moments of the past make us stronger and wiser. The present and the future, however, are ahead of us and can be under our control. This is the central message of grief processing.

Every person who comes into this world experiences an illness or difficulty during the life. RECOVERYTRSBDGR can be a part of the acceptance of bipolar disorder and a reboot focusing on the past, on the present, and on the future.

RECOVERYTRSBDGR presents a marathon achieving improvement and a new restart in life. It is not a marathon to victory, perfectionism, or the total disappearance of problems and inabilities. It is a dynamic program that continues throughout life. It is a dynamic synthesis of ways of dealing with problems and can support not only TRSBD but also other problems.

RECOVERYTRSBDGR helps patients with TRS and their families overcome the grief of a serious mental health disorder. Pharmacotherapy for TRSBD, psycho-education, individual and group cognitive behavioral therapy, and rehabilitation present actions which are committed to life and lead to advance and enhancement.

This is the best answer to suicidality, chronic disability, weakness, loss of control, and desperation. In other words, the leading reply to anxiety of death as a result of a severe mental health disorder are all the appropriate actions and interventions, which keep patients with TRSBD alive, living cells of society and protagonists in their own lives.

RECOVERYTRSBDGR is devoted to the dignity of life and offers alternative ways to dead ends.

If polypharmacy had a voice, what would it say?

The combination of many medications (8 per day) will calm you down and give you a chance to sleep better and not fight or be in a better mood. *Your mood will improve in less than 10 days and you will have very good functional outcomes. You will achieve your goals within a few months.*

What would RECOVERYTRSBDGR answer?

The researches have highlighted specific empirical data. Not many agents are needed, but maybe better combinations. *The combination of many drugs will bring you many side effects, which will create a very poor quality of life. Your health is also at risk. You need less medication and long-term psychotherapy.*

If non-evidence-based psychotherapies had a voice, what would they say?

We will implement very good therapies; we know they will help you. *Trust the instinct of psychotherapists. Since we see that they work, then there is no need to worry.*

What would RECOVERYTRSBDGR answer?

There are evidence-based psychotherapies available that can help you. *RECOVERYTRSBDGR is a combination of evidence-based pharmacotherapy and psychotherapies, whose effectiveness and efficacy has been proven in recent years.*

If resistant bipolar disorder had a voice, what would it say?

I can't sleep, I'm always tense, I eat little, I talk a lot all day, I want to spend money all the time, I misunderstand people and fight with them, and I hear voices commenting on me (mania).

I sleep all day, I can't concentrate on anything, I eat a lot, I see everything black, no one wants me, I don't want to meet anyone, I want to kill myself (depression).

I have tried most of the agents. No one can balance mania and depression so effectively. Only lithium helped me a lot. But I don't like stability.

Depression sinks me and I don't need to do anything. All attention is on me. Mania sends me sky high. I am a very important person. Of course, I prefer mania.

So mood stabilization leads me to boredom and the fact that I feel empty. My life has no meaning. I am TRSBD. I can't live without this storm!

What would RECOVERYTRSBDGR answer?

You are tired of the fact that your treatments were not effective. This led to you stopping the medication and relapsing. You prefer the manic phase because you have more energy. But this phase is self-destructive because, for example, you spend a lot of money and fight with everyone. So we will make a new beginning with the pharmacotherapy and you will take the x combination, which will improve your sleep and mood step by step.

Then we will call your family to inform them and show you a way of communication, which will improve the cohesion. They have no right to verbally abuse you, just as you should not be aggressive toward your family.

Psychotherapy will help you restructure beliefs related to depression or mania, build a program of mood-enhancing activities, and train you in relapse prevention. You will learn to recognize thoughts about your thoughts.

You have your own personality. You are not the bipolar disorder.

If grief due to TRSBD had a voice, what would it say?

I wake up and go to sleep with a big reason! Why should I have this disorder? Am I being punished for something? At the beginning, I was shocked as I was hospitalized. I am very angry, and I deny what my doctors and psychotherapists tell me. I feel very tired, I cannot sleep well, and I have a depressive mood all day. I cannot live with that. I will stop taking my pharmacotherapy, and I will wake up from a bad dream. The truth is me and my life. Everything different from that is not the truth! I will follow my instinct, and my life belongs to me.

I don't want to visit psychiatrists and psychotherapists! I don't need any treatment.

I will follow what my voices suggest; in other words, live your lives without treatment. I would like to have the freedom to do everything I want! Together with my depression and mania!

My grief for my child has deep roots and will never be uprooted! I will live a life of despair and try to find comfort in friends. There is no way out of this life other than deep grief. Anger, denial, depression, hopelessness, and pessimism. I will not be happy to see my child achieve goals. What a shame! What a misfortune!

If RECOVERYTRSBDGR had a voice, how would it respond to grief?

RECOVERYTRSBDGR will help you live with more freedom, determination, and autonomy and with a higher quality of life. Your family will have a better psycho education regarding TRSBD; you will be able to control your mood and psychotic symptoms that cause distress; you will learn to enhance your mood; you will improve your cognitive functions that lead to a better functional outcome, and finally, you will improve your ability to recognize your thoughts about thoughts.

All these strategies show how not to focus on why I have this disorder, but how I cope with it gaining more control over it! In other words, RECOVERYTRSBDGR will help you transform the grief regarding TRSBD into action for life with more hope, autonomy, creativity, determination, and activation for resources! That's real life! So keep going with your therapy with hope and discipline!

RECOVERYTRSBDGR will help you go through your grief regarding the TRSBD of your child. You will be an active partner in the therapy. You will support your child through the small changes during treatment. Yes, he/she can travel, he/she can work for a few hours, he/she can fall in love, and she/he can enjoy small, beautiful everyday moments.

If stigma had a voice, what would it say?

The TRSBD label will mark you forever and leave a mark on you. The stigma you put on yourself and what others put on you. So you will be ashamed and isolated and you will not ask for any help out of shame. You are at a dead end, and society has marginalized you. There is no chance to find a solution. You are a stigma!

If RECOVERYTRSBDGR had a voice, how would it respond to stigma?

RECOVERYTRSBDGR gives you the opportunity to get to know TRSBD better, to learn to manage it with treatments, and to be the protagonist in solving problems. That way, you won't be ashamed of anything. You will be proud of the effort you are making to deal with TRSBD. Since you know what TRSBD is and how you are treated, there is no stigma. We all have a right in life to be vulnerable and to be sick!

The best response to stigma is to act for life, communicate with others, and claim from society what belongs to us. Fear, shame, and pessimism have no place in our lives. Be yourself and improve through RECOVERYTRSBDGR.

If the cognitive perspective had a voice, what would RECOVERYTRSBDGR say?

I will help you restructure the beliefs associated with weakness and confinement (depression) and grandiosity (mania). Every day you will have a repertoire of activities, which will help you improve your mood, sleep well, and maintain your social relationships.

If the metacognitive perspective had a voice, what would RECOVERYTRSBDGR say?

You will be trained to observe thoughts about thoughts and to recognize cognitive distortions.

If the recovery perspective had a voice, what would RECOVERYTRSBDGR say?

Dr. Rakitzi and Dr. Georgila will evaluate your improvement with psychometric questionnaires (Recovery as an outcome). You, as the protagonist, will make your own evaluation of your progress every hour, every day, every week, every month, and every year. Your information is important to mental health professionals. You are a valuable partner.

The therapeutic relationship in the context of RECOVERYTRSBDGR is motivation-, resource-, and recovery-oriented. The advantages and disadvantages of every potential for change and progress will be analyzed. In other words, the therapeutic relationship is a slide to implement changes and improve the quality of life. Thus, patients play a leading role in their own lives through the model of the therapeutic relationship. The therapeutic relationship is an oasis in the desert, where the patients with TRS can rest, relax and discuss all their problems in a safe environment.

Each session of RECOVERYTRSBDGR gives the opportunity to discuss changes, either for improvements that were made or for unattainable changes. The words change and progress, improvement and achievement of goals are expressed in each session and characterize the therapeutic relationship in RECOVERYTRSBDGR.

The therapeutic relationship in RECOVERYTRSBDGR increases motivation for change and progress, which simultaneously reduces stigma. The therapeutic relationship is a protection against stigma and isolation because it mobilizes the individual toward change.

The role of the family is very important in RECOVERYTRSBDGR. The Greek family supports its children in general throughout their lives and much more when they suffer from chronic health problems, such as TRSBD. Thus, we included in RECOVERYTRSBDGR a basic cultural element of Greece: the family. Most people with TRSBD live with their families and enjoy their support. Thus, by including the family in our therapy, we make it a dynamic and decisive element of the treatment, and at the same time, we intervene in it in order to reduce the high expressed emotion toward the patients with TRSBD.

TRSBD displays a distinct category of bipolar disorder. Patients with TRSBD should distinguish between themselves and their disorder. They are not the disorder, the TRSBD. They are people with their own personalities, their own human rights for access to effective treatments, and with the potential to live a life with a better quality of life. They have the right to stand up for themselves and to be assertive toward TRSBD. But they are not their disorder. They are human beings with the potential for change and improvement!

RECOVERYTRSBDGR offers the chance to learn to cope with TRSBD, to be a protagonist in one's life and to fulfill life goals. TRSBD should not be the biggest obstacle, but a problem like all the others, and with RECOVERYTRSBDGR goal is possible. Problems should be evaluated as challenges for improvement and progress and as triggers for enhancing the learning potential of patients with TRSBD and their families. Having a chronic mental health disorder and coping with it proves that the person is very strong and resilient. It is an honor for mental health experts to meet these people and to have cooperated with them.

The value and dignity of human life are guaranteed by the Declaration of Human Rights. Every person has the right to live with dignity, to satisfy his biological and emotional needs, to work, to enjoy his life, and, in cases of illness and disability, to be able to access effective treatments. Effective treatments must be applied by specialized experts with clinical experience, who will be evaluated in terms of their scientific work. These effective treatments should reach all states of the world, especially poorer countries.

The implementation of evidence-based interventions in science to address health problems is also a key criterion for the quality of democracy in any country. The right to health, access to modern treatments, and the protection of our fellow vulnerable citizens are the basic goods of every democracy!

The protection of patients with TRSBD and their families is a basic obligation of every democratic society. It is not possible to hear that TRSBD has reached a dead end, that the only treatment is ECT, and that patients have been abused by non-evidence-based interventions and by mental health experts. If all this is happening, then what quality of democracy do we have?

What is the relationship between democracy and science? Science operates within the framework of democracy and with the rules of democracy. The rights of science stop where its obligations to others, begin. Science has an obligation to produce effective tools and treatments for patients with mental health disorders, and especially with TRSBD. Science is obliged to be subject to evaluations, and finally, it is obliged to ensure all people have access to it.

Greece has been going through a socioeconomic crisis from 2008 until today. Greece has many structural problems and does not invest enough funds in the field of health. Our program can fill a gap in the field of mental health in Greece and give the opportunity to patients with TRSBD and their families to participate at a low cost.

RECOVERYTRSBDGR was a very beautiful trip for us. The idea for this program began in 2008. This year begins our scientific acquaintance and cooperation in the framework of the implementation of evidence-based interventions for bipolar disorders. We have worked intensively all these years with cognitive-behavioral psychotherapy for bipolar disorder and CR-T the last years. This collaboration lead to need for a comprehensive program just for TRSBD, in which the family would participate, pharmacotherapy would be best combined with psychotherapy, and individual and group therapy would be combined. The combination of various forms of therapy is a better practice of the various functions and enhances socialization.

The sooner TRSBD is diagnosed, the better. The sooner the appropriate agent is administered, the better. As long as polypharmacy is avoided, the motivation for action for a better quality of life increases. The more interventions we combine, the better!

Our experience has shown that the appropriate pharmacotherapy for TRSBD needs two to three months to act initially. Psychotherapy can then begin.

The family plays a crucial role and can destroy or strengthen a positive therapeutic outcome.

Individual cognitive-behavioral psychotherapy gives the opportunity to build the therapeutic relationship and reduce suspicion. Skills are slowly practiced, negative beliefs will be restructured and positive beliefs will be strengthened.

Group therapy provides the opportunity to socialize and learn from others as well as implement programs to improve cognitive functions, social skills, and to restructure beliefs and thoughts.

The rotation of mental health specialists, the hospitalizations, suicide, and the despair of patients and their families particularly troubled us. The repeating vicious cycle had to be broken.

All the above factors led to the idea of RECOVERYTRSBDGR. Our program is a result of our clinical experience with TRSBD and its problems, the above conclusions and our willingness to find an alternative solution to break the vicious cycle of TRSBD.

The chronic and persistent suicidality of TRSBD is always difficult for the patients with TRSBD, their families, and mental health experts. The thought revolves around the end of life without alternative scenarios and exits and becomes an obsession day and night!

The grief of patients with TRSBD and their families is an immense cloud over their heads. Psychotic symptoms, depression, or mania-hypomania dominate throughout the day.

The abusive experiences of our patients with TRSBD were also painful and difficult for us. These experiences are stored in the memory, which is disturbed when stimuli recall the trauma.

The comorbidity of TRSBD with other health problems proves that patients with TRSBD need help dealing with TRSBD, so that they can also deal with other health problems.

TRSBD is associated with stigma. Patients and their families have been ashamed for many years and live in isolation. They do not dare to speak and claim their rights. They live immersed in their stigma and what society puts on them.

Stigma is a very big and fundamental problem in mental health disorders, especially in TRSBD. The person with TRSBD is heavily stigmatized through the vicious cycle of the disorders, ashamed of the problems, isolated, has many relapses and has no motivation to seek help.

Our patients and their families, our clinical experience, and all the above findings brought us to the idea of creating a structured treatment for TRSBD. Our discussions about these issues in the context of peer supervision and our concern about TRSBD led us to RECOVERYTRSBDGR. 2021 was the year of the first discussions, and today, with this book, our vision is slowly becoming a reality, and we are very grateful to Springer Nature.

The 140 sessions lay the foundation for a proper initiation in the context of pharmacotherapy, for the application of a wide range of psychotherapies, for a combination of psychotherapies and for cooperation with the family. This is how individual and group interventions are combined with all their advantages, and the vicious cycle of TRSBD can be broken.

Breaking the vicious circle of TRSBD leads to a bright light in the tunnel, with the prospect of getting out of it to see beautiful landscapes and an endless blue sea. There is a prospect in this life for something better; there is a prospect to better manage the mood symptoms and cognitive dysfunctions. All of these have a positive impact on functional outcomes and quality of life.

RECOVERYTRSBDGR can also lead to a reduction in stigma because people learn to manage their problems more comfortably by setting limits to any form of stigma. In other words, the best way to deal with stigma is to develop mental health resilience in the face of the problem, which RECOVERYTRSBDGR achieves.

The pilot application of RECOVERYTRSBDGR showed us the way to further research its effectiveness and efficacy. Patients with TRSBD built a more durable therapeutic relationship with us and improved symptoms, cognitive functions, functioning, and recovery.

The comorbidity of the TRSBD with severe personality disorders requires special attention. However, RECOVERYTRSBDGR focuses on the TRSBD and interventions—biological and psychotherapeutic—can stabilize bipolar disorder, which also stabilizes personality. Psychotherapy in the context of our program can also be indirectly linked to the schemas associated with the personality disorder. If the personality disorder is very severe, then the implementation of the Beck model of cognitive behavioral psychotherapy for personality disorders can be implemented after RECOVERYTRSBDGR.

The borderline personality disorder is very common. Many colleagues focus first on the therapy of this personality treatment. This has the risk of devaluation or a mistaken diagnosis when the main disorder is TRSBD. If the resistant TRSBD is stabilized with pharmacotherapy and psychotherapy, then this will also have an impact on the reduction of the problems that arise from the borderline personality disorder.

They felt that, for the first time in their lives, they dared to manage this traumatic situation, TRSBD. They can be in control and try daily to improve any malfunctions. They are the protagonists in their lives and in our lives.

Patients with TRSBD and families go through grief, despair, and suicidality in a constant effort to recover and reintegrate into society. They define their lives and set new goals. They are in recovery during their whole lives! This makes their lives different, vivid, and challenging, which is an important protective mechanism against suicidal risk.

The ability to repeat this treatment due to relapse is also a very important feature and advantage. They are given time and space to fall back into a secure frame.

Patients with TRSBD and their families need time to learn new things through RECOVERYTRSBDGR and try to slowly integrate them into their daily lives. The scope of our treatment is slowly generalizing to other goals, such as managing organic health problems or some kind of loss.

Mental health experts feel that through this structured program they have the time and space to implement their therapy by building a better therapeutic relationship with patients with TRSBD and their families. They have time to monitor them systematically and under all conditions. In this way, a better empathy for the sufferers will be developed.

The development of an integrative recovery-oriented program is due to many factors and, above all, a common vision for more democracy in mental health and of solving problems of chronic mental disorders with more flexibility, team spirit and long-term interventions.

The therapy of patients with TRSBD displays a very rich clinical and human experience. Without them, we would not have proceeded with the creation of this program. It is our honor to have met them, to have worked with them, and to have spent endless therapeutic hours with difficult but also pleasant moments!

The continuation of the application of RECOVERYTRSBDGR to other patients with TRSBD and their families, as well as the training of other colleagues in our program, is our first priority the next few years!

RECOVERYTRSBDGR will be evaluated in the next few years by us and other colleagues regarding effectiveness and efficacy. We will be exceptionally glad to cooperate with many colleagues from all over the world in order to implement our program. Science is universal and brings people together.

The development of a program for bipolar disorder and TRSBD resistant bipolar disorder is of particular importance because it was developed in Greece, a country which went through and is going through a socioeconomic crisis, which resulted in not creating a robust social and insurance system.

This program is dedicated to the human rights of this very sensitive group of people, who are particularly vulnerable. Democratic societies must provide the best possible treatments for these individuals.

The patient, who had a double diagnosis of TRSBD and a borderline personality disorder, wrote a letter to the TRSBD:

Dear TRSBD,

I have been diagnosed for many years with a borderline personality disorder. I was abused sexually in my 15s and since then a vicious cycle of impulsivity with substance abuse, reckless expense, alternation of partners, suicide attempts, hospitalization in all clinics in Athens, and the chronic feeling of futility has been going on! I took all the medicines for psychiatry. Cognitive-behavioral psychotherapy initially helped me manage my panic, improve my mood, and stabilize it and slowly reduce my impulsivity.

Suicide is something that is a big psychological trauma for me. I spent all my life in this situation. I have nightmares that I have been trying to die by suicide. I did not see a way out of my life or alternatives. It had nothing to do with my life!

The desire for suicide can be described as a dark tunnel without an exit! There is nothing but obsession with the next attempt. The brain gave the command on a permanent basis to do harm to myself. There was no other command! It had to change that! I was constantly on surveillance so that I wouldn't do harm to myself. It tired me a lot!

I was always asking for help! For me it was proof that I wanted to live. I want to live today. But without impulsivity and self-destruction!

Polypharmacy has created many side effects! Many health problems! I felt that I was an experiment of psychiatry! I had also participated on ECT sessions but I didn't want to carry on after five sessions. This was also one of the reasons for suicidal thoughts. If my life continued like this, it wouldnt matter at all. My family should also get rid of it.

When I made suicide attempts, I had a lot of guilt toward my mother, who has been taking care of me all these years. I wanted to report to the prosecutor all the psychiatrists who gave me a lot of drugs.

The family in Greece plays a decisive role in the care of people with mental health disorders. My mother was my support in difficult times! She accepted me under all conditions without a critical mood and always with patience and optimism that we will overcome the crisis!

I changed psychiatrists after the psychologist's recommendation. I had to be hospitalized again! The increased dose of antidepressant led to a manic episode. I stayed in the clinic for 3 months. Since then, the basic diagnosis has been TRSBD and borderline personality disorder. Lithium and clozapine helped me stop aggression, hospitalization every 6 months, and be able to calm down. Then, cognitive-behavioral psychotherapy helped me better stabilize my mood.

Grieving the many hospitalizations and multiple agents in the context of polypharmacy I received that didn't help is something that plagues me to this day. Why did I waste so much time? Why did I suffer so much in my life?

The difficulties started with my sexual abuse and continued for many years until I met Dr. Georgila and Dr. Rakitzi who contributed to my stabilization and reintegration into society. Looking back is always difficult. The present and the future are much better.

Dear RECOVERYTRSBDGR,

Dr. Rakitzi and Dr. Georgila invited me to participate in this treatment and it was something different from the well-known cognitive-behavioral psychotherapy. The duration of the 140 sessions, my parents' participation, and the combination of individual and group therapy with the application of various modern specialized therapies mobilized the desire for life. I have restructured my negative beliefs, strengthened my positive beliefs, and improved my quality of life. I can control my mood swings and have found a new meaning in life.

I am a mother and that gives me even greater responsibility to be as healthy as possible and more grounded in reality. Treatment has helped me become a mother and withstand the difficulties of life! My mother also played a decisive role in that. I'm glad I have given her the joy of becoming a grandmother!

I understood that my main problem is TRSBD and not borderline personality disorder. The regulation of bipolar disorder has also equalized my impulsivity. My personality, in other words, is more stable.

I feel grateful for this treatment. Clozapine with lithium and long-term psychotherapy have helped me feel useful in society and my family.

I was in grief for a long time. Why it so difficult all these years to make the right diagnosis and to get the right agent? Why should my life be in danger so many times?

Polypharmacy could have led me to death! This finding, after so many years, led me to appreciate every day and every minute of my life! I am grateful to live!

I would also like to send a message: People suffering from chronic mental disorders have the right to access effective therapies without exploiting polypharmacy. Polypharmacy creates more problems and can cause many organic health problems.

But my life continues to improve today and that matters. There are no dead ends in our lives! This is for sure! I can now coexist peacefully with the TRSBD and regulate my thinking and behavior every day!

An internal self-regulation mechanism has been installed after RECOVERYTRSBDGR.

Dr. Georgila's letter to TRSBD,

Dear TRSBD,

Bipolar disorder and TRSBD were and are for me, a daily routine of my work. I can't do without it. The TRSBD is greater in percentage than we imagined.

Your vicious cycle of suicidal risk, relapses, discontinuation of agents, and constant changes of mental health experts has tired and saddened me many times.

Worst of all was polypharmacy, with many side effects for patients with TRSBD. But I learned to deal with you. I have been giving antidepressants, mood stabilizers, and antipsychotic agents from the beginning, depending on the individual's problems, which is very effective for TRSBD. I also trained many mental health experts in it. So there is a way to deal with TRSBD. But we need new agents for TRSBD. I also propose long-term psychotherapy.

The alternations of depression and mania, or depression and hypomania, are very tiring for sufferers. The cyclothymic disorder with mood swings that happen within the same day is also very tiring. The adjustment of medication should be done every month, and in periods of crisis, the follow-up should be more systematic.

Clinical psychiatrists can deal with you building from beginning a therapeutic relationship with the prospect of maintaining it over time. Psycho-education for TRSBD and appropriate biological and psychotherapeutic interventions can set boundaries and structure in such a difficult and chronic disorder.

I was shocked many years ago by the story of a young man with TRSBD, who nearly died from polypharmacy. The dual trauma of TRSBD and abuse with the agents was in front of me in every session. I couldn't avoid it. I helped this young man quite effectively, and I also suggested cognitive behavioral psychotherapy.

The stigma of TRSBD is a very big problem. People remained untreated and isolated for many years because of their shame. Thus precious time was lost.

I am optimistic about the future of pharmacotherapy regarding TRSBD. There are also very effective psychotherapies available.

Dr. Georgila's letter to RECOVERYTRSBDGR,

Dear RECOVERYTRSBDGR,

The idea of developing a therapy for TRSBD gave me great joy and optimism. RECOVERYTRSBDGR makes it possible, step by step, to build a therapeutic relationship of trust and security. Pharmacotherapy is discussed from the first moment, and all the difficulties of the past are analyzed. We are making a new beginning with the agents.

The family will be included. This is very important because family plays a crucial role in the lives of patients with TRSBD. Individual and group cognitive-behavioral psychotherapy are being implemented in the long term. This gives us the opportunity to arm our patients with the skills to reintegrate into society more quickly. Thus, stigma is reduced, and functionality and self-confidence are improved.

RECOVERYTRSBDGR has relaxed me. Patients with TRSBD were in long-term treatment, and the multiple hospitalizations and suicidal risk were interrupted.

The dynamic and long-term implementation of RECOVERYTTRSBDGR gives hope and a way out for patients with TRSBD and their families.

Thank you for giving me the opportunity to help my patients in a structured and long-term way. This fills me with optimism and gives me the possibility of multiple interventions over a long period of time. 140 sessions are enough to solve past problems and make a new beginning in life.

Dr. Rakitzi's letter to TRSBD,

Dear TRSBD,

I was confronted with TRSBD years ago in my private practice. At that time, I didn't have enough clinical experience. I was scared and referred the patient to the hospital. I am saddened by the stigma you leave on patients with TRSBD and their families, their grief, and your complexity. The stigma among these patients is very large and deep. They stay for many years without treatment because they are ashamed.

Today, I feel safer with TRSBD. I know the difficulties, how I have to increase their motivation, and that suicide is the first priority in the treatment. I also know that the appropriate combination of agents is very effective for patients with TRSBD.

The first thing that strikes me in the history of a person with TRSBD is the many and rapid changes of agents, with the argument that the agents are not effective. When I hear such a story, the first thing I do is to immediately contact the psychiatrist and understand what has happened. What I can definitely do against you is a dynamic long-term, effective psychotherapy.

The grief and stigma you leave in patients with TRSBD and their families is outrageous! These two traumas contribute to the isolation from society, reduce the possibility of seeking help, and increase the chance that they will never get out of this vicious circle. Misery and introversion!

Your vicious cycle makes me angry, saddens me, and, at the same time, motivates me to break it psychotherapeutically. The priority is the right pharmacotherapy, and after the patient is stabilized, psychotherapies can be applied. There are ways to deal with it.

There are no dead ends in this life! I challenge you to come and see how one can better regulate mood by encouraging individual responsibility in patients with TRSBD.

Dr. Rakitzi's letter to RECOVERYTRSBDGR,

Dear RECOVERYTRSBDGR,

I am very happy to participate in the development of this recovery-oriented treatment program. It is a systematic program that combines pharmacotherapy and individual and group psychotherapy. This variety of interventions can manage the complex problems of TRSBD at all levels.

Improvements in symptoms, cognitive functions and thinking lead to improvements in functional outcomes and quality of life. Chronic grief turns into action for life, and the stigma is replaced by the confidence to accept and defend myself as I am!

I am optimistic with you that we will powerfully help many patients with TRSBD. We will make it. If anything counts in this life, it is action for life.

This action also makes sense to me because I can effectively help my vulnerable fellow citizens with more than 67% disability.

What I love about therapy is its ability to holistically intervene with suicidal risk, grief, and stigma. Acting for life washes away all that misery and isolation. The stigma in particular is deeply rooted in TRSBD since it appears from the first moment problems manifest and from the first acute psychotic episode. It's like a trauma!

RECOVERYTRSBDGR gives us the possibility to break the vicious cycle of TRSBD by reducing the stigma and grief and strengthening the relationships with the family and the personal development of the patient with TRSBD. Thank you for this beautiful trip.

I will continue this effort with you at every opportunity. This is how we will reduce the suicidal risk of these people to a minimum, and we will integrate them into society.

The most important thing is that you give perspective to people's lives with dignity, respect and hope.

RECOVERYTRSBDGR will be evaluated in the future in terms of its effectiveness and efficacy in clinical practice. Time will highlight its advantages and disadvantages.

RECOVERYTRSBDGR fills me with optimism, gives me energy, and reminds me that goal-directed and structured treatment can lead to desired results. It takes persistence and patience,

All the best for all of us!

A large percentage of bipolar disorder belongs to TRSBD. This led to the need to create a specialized program for TRSBD. This category is the most difficult and needs specific therapeutic strategies. It is the category that creates frustration and hopelessness.

The TRSBD carries a very heavy load. They have a very deep stigma and isolate themselves from society. They are overwhelmed and do not ask for help from the experts. Interfamily relationships are often disturbed. Their grief, which manifests itself in psychotic symptoms, is also very deep and lasting. They often face traumas, such as physical, sexual, and psychological abuse. These traumas reinforce grief as well as stigma.

The above load presupposes a structured and evidence-based treatment of TRSBD. The therapeutic relationship combined with interventions can be a springboard to deal with the disorder and then the rest, such as trauma, grief, and stigma. RECOVERYTRSBDGR is a long-term action for life that gives the right to leave with dignity, pride and assertiveness.

RECOVERYTRSBDGR gives TRSBD a chance. It reduces frustration, increases hope, and intervenes on all levels. It respects the patients with TRSBD and their families. RECOVERYTRSBDGR protects against abuse and constitutes a democratic framework for intervention. Its duration is long term, and this can be tiring, but on the other hand, TRSBD is only treated long-term and with a combination of interventions.

RECOVERYTRSBDGR gives a basic message of life in TRSBD, but also in any chronic mental health disorder. There are problems and obstacles with malfunctions in everyday life. There is the grief, the stigma, and the trauma. But there is also a structured response for action to life.

RECOVERYTRSBDGR gives inspiration to patients with TRSBD because it focuses on their problems by accepting them and changing their life conditions.

RECOVERYTRSBDGR confronts action for life against misery, powerlessness, and vulnerability. It inspires mental health experts, patients with TRSBD and their families to be cohesive, optimistic, motivation-, recovery-, and resource-oriented against misery, vulnerability and weakness.

Mental health experts have a long history of studies, training, and retraining. The initial stages of dealing with mental disorders entail the need for much observation, the acquisition of clinical experience, the need for supervision with a supervisor, supervision with colleagues and further training.

The completion of the above first cycle opens the second cycle, which is related to the application of acquired knowledge and deepening in clinical experience. The second cycle opens a third cycle, in which the need to develop something new and implement it over time is created! This is how it happened with RECOVERYTRSBDGR. A third cycle was opened, which involves the development of a new program that will be implemented more systematically in the coming years and whose effectiveness and efficacy will be investigated.

This third cycle is opened by the mental health experts after internal mental processes and, at the same time, as a result of the supervision. The following processes are carried out for every mental health disorder, but especially for TRSBD:

The empathy of mental health experts results in greater compassion for the problems of TRSBD patients and their families.

The long-term implementation of effective treatments in these patients leads to an analysis of the advantages and disadvantages of available treatments and what may be missing. This gap will be filled by the creation of a new program.

The biological vulnerability of patients with TRSBD makes interventions even more difficult. All the agents and the available psychotherapies have been tried many times and we go back again, to the relapse. This raises the concerns of mental health professionals and they are looking for interventions that will continuously increase motivation and be long term.

Opinions on the implementation of long-term evidence-based programs in mental health differ. One could argue that long-term treatments tire and bring people face-to-face with their vulnerabilities. Does this fatigue lead them to the opposite results? Should we leave them alone? Monthly psychiatric follow-up is sufficient.

There is no need for psychotherapy. Psychotherapy will increase grief, which one should repress and not engage with. Let's try to help people have a good time in their lives, as long as they have good adherence to pharmacotherapy.

The answer to the above arguments is that this avoidance strategy will lead to the deterioration of the condition of patients with TRSBD, they will not be given the opportunity to be trained in a structured and safe framework to deal with their problems, and thus the importance of medication compliance. This will have the effect of not building the appropriate resilience against the difficulties of everyday life and increasing the possibility of self-destructive and hetero-destructive behaviors. Short-term fatigue from a systemic treatment will lead to greater safety in the long term.

A new therapeutic program, which is intended for chronic mental health disorders and especially for TRSBD, must have the following characteristics:

- *To focus on the main therapeutic goals in bipolar disorder: reducing depressive, manic and hypomanic symptoms, improving cognitive functions, quality of life, and functionality.*
- *To include psycho-education of the family.*
- *To be applied long-term and to increase the motivation for life.*
- *To have the possibility of repetition in case of needs and a negative result from the first application.*
- *At the same time, research should be conducted on its effectiveness and efficacy in clinical practice conditions.*
- *To reduce the stigma that turns patients and their families away from the treatments.*
- *To give an outlet to the chronic grief of patients and their families. May grief be turned into action for living meaningful.*
- *To enhance resilience in the present and in the future.*

The stigma of patients and their families leads to hopelessness, isolation, depression, increased feelings of shame, and suicidal risk. The stigma comes from the sufferers themselves but also from society. Stigma is very strong and negatively affects adherence to treatment. It breaks up treatments and therapeutic relationships, reduces life expectancy, and makes everyday life and quality of life difficult. Action against stigma is ongoing and should begin immediately. Action against stigma is a living mechanism of a democratic society.

Grief in the face of a chronic mental disorder is a normal reaction that has been hidden for many years in the souls of patients and their families. Why would I have TRSBD so early that I can't complete things, can't study properly, work and enjoy my life without the storms of my emotions? Why me;

This process must be processed in order to gradually end up in the acceptance and restart based on the new facts of life. Life must be based on the realistic facts and capabilities of the individual. Patients and their families have the right to grieve, despair, and mourn as much as they need to. The expression of grief reduces the possibility of the establishment of a chronic, resistant depression, which can increase the suicidal risk. Processing grief releases energy and gives new perspective for a fresh start.

The cognitive perspective relates to one's thoughts and beliefs about oneself, others, and the future. In other words, how various events and situations are interpreted which has affected the emotional and behavioral level.

The metacognitive perspective focuses on thoughts about thoughts. So the person takes a mental distance from his interpretations and thoughts and revises some things! Thus, it re-evaluates situations through a new synthesis of information.

The recovery perspective as an outcome and as a process, as discussed in this book, highlights the importance of collaboration between mental health professionals and patients with TRSBD and their families. Recovery will be evaluated from both sides, which will complement each other.

A comprehensive program for TRSBD, which combines evidence-based interventions whose effectiveness and efficacy have been established, gives sufferers and their families the opportunity to participate in as many treatments as possible. So this is of great therapeutic benefit because the program focuses on improving the core problems of TRSBD, including functional outcome, recovery, and quality of life. A comprehensive program will combine individual and group therapy and provide additional treatments such as couple therapy and family intervention.

An integrative program will take into account and provide intervention to address the stigma of TRSBD as well as the processing of grief as a result of living with a chronic mental health disorder. Stigma and grief lead to isolation, depression, a lack of hope, and taking individual responsibility for problems. Thus, the years go by, and opportunities to participate in modern and effective treatments are not taken advantage of.

A comprehensive program should lead to increased mental health resilience.

All the above elements are taken into account in RECOVERYTRSBDGR. Our model slowly guides the person with TRSBD and their family through the combination of effective interventions at the individual and group level, from weakness, vulnerability, suspicion, depression, confinement, stigma, and grief to taking responsibility, problem- solving, autonomy, hope, and action for life.

RECOVERYTRSBDGR contributes to resilience. Resilience is the ability to adapt and deal with difficult situations in which the limits of patients with chronic mental disorders, especially with TRSBD and their families are tested. Resilience is the result of effective treatments aimed at recovery. Our model follows this specific path and activates all existing possibilities for improvement, even if they are few due to the difficult situation.

Recovery activates the resources that lead to changes and transformation and is evaluated by the mental health experts (recovery as an outcome) and the patients with TRSBD and their families (recovery as a process). It is the ultimate goal of any psychotherapy. Resilience presents the result of the recovery process and is always a filter, which increases resistance to difficulties and adaptation to new circumstances in life.

Mental health recovery and resilience is like a loving married couple. Difficulties lead them to implement effective management strategies and solve problems. Cohesiveness and resistance to difficulties builds resilience and make them stronger, energetic, and optimistic about the future. They are the real protagonists in their lives.

Below is a dialogue between resilience and recovery:

Res: Good morning. Today I was thinking about how the years have passed. We have been together for 30 years in difficult and happy moments.

Rec: Indeed! How did the time pass like this? We have been through a lot together, and this fills us with pride!

I taught us to deal with difficult times, depression, mania-hypomania, and problems in functioning. I improved our functional outcome and our quality of life. We face our everyday life better. I boosted our confidence by focusing on what we could do even better. We evaluate every day our progress and our difficulties and we are the protagonists of our lives.

Res: You are absolutely right. I, in turn, tried to put a filter on us so that, on the one hand, the application of everything we have learned is automated, and on the other hand, we withstand the stress and the difficulties by continuing the efforts with hope and optimism. Difficulties are for us a driving force for improvement and for more endurance. Difficulties are a compass for us to find new ways of managing our everyday life. Life without difficulties would be very monotonous and would not give us the opportunity to discover new ways of managing TRSBD.

In other words, recovery and resilience are the two main axes of any evidence-based pharmacotherapy and psychotherapy. They are also the two main axes of our own program.

RECOVERYTRSBDGR can strengthen the claim, that is, the ability to claim the rights, to ensure a greater quality of life and a better future without forgetting my obligations to others.

Our model can protect our vulnerable fellow citizens and their families and help them assert their rights by achieving more goals. Our model improves the relationship between patients with TRSBD and their families by creating a context of cooperation and respect. Abuse has no place in this model. Thus, people are dynamic elements of society that claim a better place in this society.

Scientists must create the right conditions within democracies so that those suffering from chronic mental health disorders are protected and empowered. This makes scientists key protectors of a resilient democracy.

The value and dignity of human life is protected by European Community law. It is the highest good for all people around the world. The implementation of evidence-based treatments for chronic mental disorders and TRSBD leads to reintegration into society in various areas, such as work, housing and leisure. If there is a balance in these areas, then the protection of the value and dignity of human life is a given.

Thus mental health experts are evaluated as a whole if, through their interventions, they protect the dignity of human life. This is a sacred, lifelong goal that gives even greater meaning to the lives of mental health professionals, and patients with chronic mental health disorders, and their families.

Our thoughts will always be with those who suffer from TRSBD and who lost their lives because they did not get into a structured evidence-based therapeutic context. But our thinking will also be about patients with TRSBD, who cannot have access to modern therapies because they live in very poor countries.

Poverty is one of the biggest factors in the deterioration of mental health disorders and deprives people of access to modern treatments. Scientists are obliged to help poor countries implement modern treatments for chronic mental health disorders.

The development of new therapeutic programs for TRSBD and research for their effectiveness and efficacy require funding and long-term research implementation!

Organic and mental health is essential parts that determine human functionality. It is the main core of life. Mental health is a driving force for life, for its evolution and for achieving every goal. Evidence-based pharmacotherapy and psychotherapy strengthen mental health, which in turn has a positive effect on one's organic health.

Pharmacotherapy ensures the necessary balance for brain neurotransmitters, which regulates cognitive functions, emotion, and behavior, and overall functional outcome, and quality of life.

Psychotherapy is stored in the brain as a learning mechanism for processing and reacting to the stimuli of everyday life, which improves daily quality of life, functional outcomes, and systematically strengthens expectations for the future. Recovery as a process by patients with TRSBD and their families renews this learning mechanism with new information and corrects any errors.

The combination of evidence-based pharmacotherapy and psychotherapy leads to a restart of the whole life. Many problems are solved and new paths are opened to achieve new goals. This new phase of life requires adjustment and a new restart. Patients with TRSBD are challenged to consider the advantages and disadvantages of these changes. They may end up having to be more functional in their lives than they thought. This is something very positive, but at the same time it also requires a new phase of adaptation.

Evidence-based psychotherapy is, in other words, a new mindset, a new philosophy of life that leaves behind all the mistakes and so the person proceeds with new and safer data. The effective combination of evidence-based pharmacotherapy and psychotherapy becomes the basic life compass for the present and the future. All life decisions are filtered through this new learning mechanism, which leaves its mark throughout life.

A new therapeutic program is born, just like a child. Waiting for the birth of the child is full of joy and optimism for the future. There will be pleasant and unpleasant moments in this child's life. What is needed for the child to be trained in durability, resilience and the ability to face difficult situations by coming out more of any difficulty and making a new restart! So is the RECOVERYTRSBDGR!

The relationship with the child is maintained forever and we monitor its development over time. This development will go through an evaluation, and measures will be taken to improve and facilitate the child's life and finally the child needs love, acceptance, and stability in his or her life.

RECOVERYTRSBDGR meets the criteria of a recovery-oriented therapy. It focuses on evidence-based therapeutic goals of TRSBD, provides individual and group intervention, enables family education, and sends an optimistic message in the context of mental health: TRSBD can be managed in a structured manner and long term.

In other words, there are solutions, as long as mental health experts make a long-term commitment to implementing evidence-based treatments. We accompany patients with TRSBD and their families throughout their lives. This presupposes on the part of mental health experts a sense of responsibility, endurance, an appropriate value system, and lifelong learning.

We wish you a nice trip RECOVERYTRSBDGR and we hope to inspire many of our colleagues all over the world! Time will show if RECOVERYTRSBDGR completes its journey and fulfill the basic goals of a recovery-oriented therapy. We are very happy to make available to the scientific community a new, modern, and recovery-oriented therapy for the patients with TRSBD and their families.

Competing Interests The authors have no conflicts of interest to declare that are relevant to the content of this chapter.

Ethical Approval Our case studies follow the ethical standards of the 1964 Declaration of Helsinki. Informed consent to publish was obtained from individual participants.